# The Complete New

# NOOM

## Diet Cookbook 2023

### Quick and Easy Healthy fresh Recipes for Weight Loss and Healthy Lifestyle

## Norma R. Ansley

# Table of Content

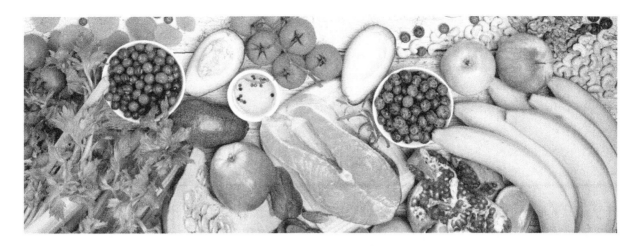

## CHAPTER 1: NOOM DIET

# Introduction

Noom promises to stop dieting and help people achieve long-lasting weight and fitness goals. According to Noom's website, Noom claims it is the "last weight-loss plan you'll ever require." Noom doesn't tell you what to eat or how to exercise. It uses psychological principles that help you to develop healthy habits to lose weight.

Noom will show you daily calories after you fill out your goals. You'll also find information on how you can improve your eating habits and workouts. It uses a color-coded system that categorizes more than a million food items according to their nutritional density. Some critics claim that the daily calorie limit is too low. Food labeling can also trigger disordered food intake, particularly for those with a history of eating disorders.

Noom's long-term, holistic approach to health allows people to shift their perspective and approach weight reduction differently. Noom shows people how to change their mindsets about weight and how to understand the importance and impact of exercise and nutrition.

# What is Noom?

Noom's primary message is that the program is psychologically based. This means that you will not only become healthier but also build habits that will sustain you throughout your life. It's easier to think of yourself as changing your habits to make you more like your best self rather than abandoning your existing lifestyle and starting a new one. The Noom diet is based on evidence-based information, cognitive behavior coaches, simple tracking tools and an easy-to-use interface.

# What is the Noom diet?

The Noom diet, which is psychology-based, promotes balance. The diet divides food into three categories: red, yellow, or green. The best foods are green; yellow foods are more nutritious, and red foods have the highest calories. Your ideal diet should consist mostly of green foods and some yellow foods with a small amount of red food.

These categories serve more as a guideline than a set of rules. "If you exceed your Red food allowance for the day but keep within your daily calorie limit, there are no repercussions other than seeing your target ceiling on the bar chart.

Noom reminds users that red foods aren't exempted in any way. The color system doubles up as a guide for portion sizes. Dessert is possible, as most of your meals were primarily green and yellow. We have the science to explain the diet to you if you are curious.

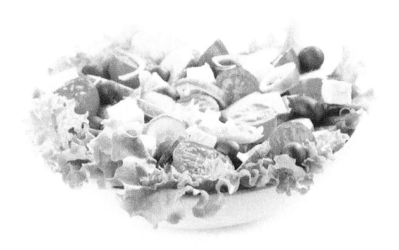

## CHAPTER 2: BREAKFAST

## Fruit Delight

Prep time: 15 minutes

Cook time: 0 minutes

Serving: 6

### Ingredients

- 250 grams strawberries
- 1 apple
- 1 pear
- 1 kiwi
- 200 ml heavy whipping cream
- 1 tablespoon of powdered sugar
- 1 teaspoon of vanilla extract
- Cinnamon powder

### Instructions

1. Remove the stem from the strawberries and wash them. Place the strawberries into a blender. Blend on high until you have a creamy mixture.

2. Whip the cream in a bowl with 1 tablespoon of powdered sugar. Add the vanilla extract to make stiff peaks. Mix in the ground strawberries. Fold gently with a spatula.
3. Wash the fruit and peel it. Chop the fruit into small pieces. Mix the cream with the fruit. Let cool for around an hour. Remove from refrigerator, sprinkle cinnamon and serve.

# Oatmeal Blueberry Pancakes

Prep time: 3 minutes

Cook time: 7 minutes

Serving: 1

## Ingredients

- 1/2 cup of oats
- 2 tablespoons of yogurt
- 1/3 teaspoon of baking soda
- 1/3 teaspoon of baking powder
- 1 teaspoon of vanilla
- 1 egg
- 1/3 cup of blueberries
- 1 tablespoon of maple syrup
- coconut oil for the pan

## Instructions

1. Blend all ingredients in a blender except for the blueberries. If you are using ground oats, you can use a hand blender with a bowl or just one bowl with a fork.
2. Heat coconut oil on medium heat. Pour the batter into a small-sized pan and cook. Blueberries can be used to top the pancake batter.
3. When the edges are smooth, and bubbles appear, use the spatula to work around the edges and flip the pancakes. Continue this process until you run out.
4. Serve immediately with maple syrup, honey, and additional blueberries.

# Baby Spinach Omelet

Prep time: 5 minutes

Cook time: 10 minutes

Serving: 1

## Ingredients

- 2 eggs
- 1 cup of torn baby spinach leaves
- 1 ½ tablespoons of grated Parmesan cheese
- ¼ teaspoon of onion powder
- ⅛ teaspoon of ground nutmeg
- salt and pepper as needed

## Instructions

1. Mix eggs in a bowl. Add baby spinach and Parmesan cheese. Season the dish with salt, pepper, nutmeg and onion powder.
2. Spray a small skillet with cooking spray, and heat on medium heat. When the skillet is warm, add the egg mixture. Cook for 3 minutes. Continue cooking for 2 to 3 more minutes by flipping the eggs over with a spatula.
3. Turn down the heat and cook for 2 to 3 more minutes or until the omelet is cooked to your liking.

# Avocado Toast

Prep time: 3 minutes

Cook time: 2 minutes

Serving: 1

## Ingredients

- 1 slice of bread
- ½ ripe avocado
- Pinch of salt

## Instructions

1. Toast your bread slice until it is golden brown.
2. The pit should be removed from the avocado. Scoop out the flesh with a large spoon. You can place the flesh in a bowl. Then, use a fork to mash it. Mix in a pinch of salt. If you like, add more salt.
3. Spread avocado on toast. Enjoy the toast as-is, or top it with extras.

# Scrambled Eggs and Tomatoes

Prep time: 5 minutes

Cook time: 20 minutes

Serving: 4

## Ingredients

- 4 eggs
- 4 tomatoes
- 4 tablespoons of cooking oil
- some pinches salt

## Instructions

1. Place the eggs in a bowl. Mix the eggs with salt.
2. In a large saucepan, heat enough oil to fry the eggs. Once they are 70% done, transfer them to a plate and set them aside.
3. Preparing tomatoes: Chop and slice tomatoes into small pieces.
4. Add the remaining oil to the pan. Once the oil has been absorbed, add the chopped tomatoes and stir. Season with salt. Let it simmer for 2 minutes or until the tomatoes shrink, and the juices start to come out.
5. Put the eggs back in the pan. Please give it a quick stir to ensure that the tomato juice reaches the eggs.

# Strawberry Mango Smoothie

Prep time: 3 minutes

Cook time: 2 minutes

Serving: 2

## Ingredients

- 2 cups of frozen sliced strawberries
- 1 1/2 cups of frozen mango pieces
- 1/2 cup of chopped carrots or baby carrots
- 1 1/2 cups of unsweetened almond milk
- 1 tablespoon of freshly squeezed lemon juice

## Instructions

1. All ingredients should be placed in a blender, including strawberries, carrots (mango), almond milk, and lemon zest.
2. Blend until smooth. Enjoy immediately.

# Grilled Peanut Butter and Banana Sandwich

Prep time: 2 minutes

Cook time: 10 minutes

Serving: 1

## Ingredients

- cooking spray
- 2 tablespoons of peanut butter
- 2 slices whole wheat bread
- 1 banana, sliced

## Instructions

1. Cook the griddle or skillet on medium heat. Once it is hot, spray it with cooking spray. One tablespoon of peanut butter should be spread on each bread slice. Place banana slices on the peanut butter side of one slice. Cover the other

with another slice and press down. For about 2 minutes on each side, fry the sandwich.

# Raspberry Lime Smoothie

Prep time: 3 minutes

Cook time: 2 minutes

Serving: 2

## Ingredients

- 2 cups of hulled raspberries, blueberries
- 1 banana
- 1/2 cup of orange juice
- 1 tablespoon of lime
- 1/2 cup of crushed ice
- 2 mint leaves or lime wedges garnish

## Instructions

1. Blend all ingredients in a blender until smooth.
2. Mix in 2 glasses. Garnish with a lime wedge or mint leaves.

# Healthy Breakfast Burrito

Prep time: 10 minutes

Cook time: 20 minutes

Serving: 4

## Ingredients

- 4 oz. red potatoes, cubed
- 4 Sugarhouse Maple Breakfast Chicken Sausages
- 1/2 cup of diced yellow onion
- 1/2 cup of diced red bell pepper
- 2 cups of spinach, chopped
- 4 large eggs

- 8 egg whites
- 1 teaspoon of garlic powder
- 1/2 teaspoon of onion powder
- Salt + Pepper as needed
- 4 large tortillas

## Instructions

1. Cook the potatoes in a large skillet coated with nonstick cooking spray for about 3 to 5 minutes or until softened. Add the chopped chicken sausage to the skillet along with the bell pepper and onion. Cook for another minute, then add the spinach. After the veggies are tender and the sausage is browned, you can add eggs, whites, and seasonings.
2. Place 1/4 cup of the egg mixture in each tortilla. Add any toppings that you like. Place the filling on the tortilla sides and roll up, making sure to tuck in the edges.
3. Spray the skillet with cooking spray, and turn the heat to medium. Once the skillet is hot, add the burritos seam-side down. Cover the skillet and cook the burritos for 3 minutes. Turn the burritos upside down and cook for a few more minutes, covered. Serve warm.
4. You can make your burritos ahead of time by wrapping them tightly in plastic wrap, refrigerating them, and then cooking. Wrap leftover burritos in foil for reheating. Bake in a 350F oven for 15 minutes.

# Customizable Microwave Eggs

Prep time: 2 minutes

Total time: 2 minutes

Serving: 1

## Ingredients

### Base Recipe:

- 4 egg whites for higher protein
- 2 tablespoons of unsweetened almond milk
- salt and pepper as needed
- Optional Add In's
- 1/8 cup of broccoli rice

- 1/2 teaspoon of garlic powder
- 1/2 teaspoon of thyme

## Instructions

1. Olive oil sprays a 12- to the 15-oz. mug.
2. Add eggs, milk and salt. Mix until the yolks are broken down and the eggs become fluffy. As desired, add optional add-ins. Mix well.
3. Heat the mug in the microwave for 30 seconds, stirring occasionally.
4. Eggs can be cooked in a matter of 1-2 minutes.
5. Take the microwave out of your kitchen and enjoy.

# Scrambled Eggs with Cheese

Prep time: 2 minutes

Cook time: 3 minutes

Serving: 1

## Ingredients

- 2 eggs
- ¼ cup of cheddar cheese, grated
- ½ teaspoon of olive oil
- Salt and pepper as needed
- 1 slice of whole grain bread

## Instructions

1. Place the butter or oil in a frying pan on medium heat.
2. Mix the eggs in a bowl. Use a fork to beat them quickly.
3. Make the cheese by grating it and preparing it.
4. Place the eggs in a frying pan.
5. Add the cheese to the top.
6. Once the eggs are inserted from the sides to the middle with a spatula, they will begin solidifying quickly.
7. You can do this several times.
8. This takes very little time. The idea is that you will have soft, lightly-cooked fresh eggs. It isn't easy to undercook eggs, but easy to overcook them. You will only need to cook the egg for 2-3 minutes.

9. You're done when the egg is completely dry. Remove from heat quickly and place on a plate, preferably with some hot, unbuttered bread.
10. Salt and pepper to your liking. Done!

# Apple Banana Nut Oatmeal

Prep time: 2 minutes

Cook time: 5 minutes

Serving: 2

## Ingredients

- 1 cup of skim milk
- 1 cup of water
- 1 teaspoon of vanilla
- 1 teaspoon of cinnamon
- ¼ teaspoon of nutmeg
- 1 pinch of sea salt
- 1 cup of old-fashioned oats
- 1 banana
- 1 apple
- 2 tablespoons of flaxseed meal
- 2 tablespoons of walnuts

## Instructions

1. Mix milk, water and vanilla in a saucepan over medium heat. Add a pinch of salt.
2. Bring to a boil slowly and then add the oats and banana.
3. Bring mixture to a boil, then reduce heat to low and simmer for 5 minutes.
4. Mix well and add walnuts and flax during the final minutes.
5. When oatmeal reaches the desired consistency, serve.

# Scrambled eggs with basil, spinach & tomatoes

Prep time: 5 minutes

Cook time: 5 minutes

Serving: 2

## Ingredients

- 1 tablespoon of olive oil, plus 1 teaspoon of
- 3 tomatoes, halved
- 4 large eggs
- 4 tablespoons of natural bio yogurt
- ⅓ small pack of basil, chopped
- 175g baby spinach, dried well

## Instructions

1. Place the tomatoes in a large, non-stick pan. Heat 1 teaspoon of oil and then cook them, cut side down, on medium heat. While they cook, mix the yogurt with 2 tablespoons of water, lots of black pepper, and the basil in a small bowl.
2. Transfer the tomatoes to plates. Mix the spinach into the pan. While the eggs are cooking, stir the spinach a few more times.
3. Heat the remaining oil in a non-stick skillet on medium heat. Once the eggs are scrambled, add the egg mixture. Stir occasionally. Spread the spinach onto plates. Top with scrambled eggs.

# Avocado and Egg

Prep time: 3 minutes

Cook time: 7 minutes

Serving: 1

## Ingredients

- 1 Avocado Peeled, sliced into 8 wedges
- 1 Egg poached
- 8 stalks of Baby asparagus roasted
- 1 tablespoon of Balsamic vinegar
- Black pepper fresh ground

## Instructions

1. Preheat oven to 350°F. To coat the stalks, place baby asparagus on a small baking sheet. Place the stalks on a baking sheet and drizzle some balsamic vinegar. Roll them in it.
2. Bring a small saucepan of water to a boil. Then, bake the asparagus for about 5 to 7 minutes. Be careful not to leave it in there too long. The egg should be poached for 3 minutes.
3. While the asparagus and egg are in the oven, slice and wedge the avocado.
4. Arrange the asparagus on top of the avocado wedges, then place the poached eggs in the middle. If desired, garnish with fresh ground black pepper or additional balsamic vinegar.

# Quinoa Breakfast Scramble

Prep time: 10 minutes

Cook time: 10 minutes

Serving: 4

## Ingredients

- 1 Tablespoon of olive oil
- 1 cup of tomatoes, diced
- 2 cups of fresh baby spinach
- 1 cup of Central Market Organic Quinoa, cooked

- 4 large eggs, beaten
- 1/4 cup of herb Parmesan Cheese

## Instructions

1. On medium heat, heat olive oil in a large skillet. Cook the tomatoes for 3-4 minutes.
2. Add the spinach to the pan and cook until tender and most liquid has evaporated.
3. Continue to cook for 2 minutes.
4. Mix in the beaten eggs. Cook, stirring, until firm.
5. Divide the bowls among four bowls and sprinkle cheese on top.

# Tofu Scramble

Prep time: 10 minutes

Total time: 10 minutes

Serving: 2

## Ingredients

- 1 tablespoon of olive oil
- 16-oz. block firm tofu
- 2 tablespoons of nutritional yeast
- 1/2 teaspoon of salt, or more as needed
- 1/4 teaspoon of turmeric
- 1/4 teaspoon of garlic powder
- 2 tablespoons of non-dairy milk, unsweetened and unflavored

## Instructions

1. Place the olive oil in a saucepan over medium heat. With a potato mashing tool or a fork, mash the tofu in the pan. You can also use your hands to crumble the tofu into the pan. Cook the tofu for about 3-4 mins, stirring often, until the water is almost gone.
2. Next, add the nutritional yeast and salt. Continue to stir for 5 minutes.
3. Mix the non-dairy dairy milk in a saucepan. Serve immediately with sliced avocados, hot sauce, parsley or toast.

# Zucchini Bread Oatmeal

Prep time: 5 minutes

Cook time: 8 minutes

Serving: 2

## Ingredients

### *For the oatmeal:*

- 14-oz. light coconut milk
- 2/3 cup of gluten-free rolled oats
- 1 cup of packed finely grated zucchini
- 2 tablespoons of chia seeds
- 1/2 to 1 teaspoon of cinnamon, as needed
- 1/4 teaspoon of freshly grated nutmeg
- 1 1/2 tablespoons of pure maple syrup
- Small pinch of fine sea salt
- 1 teaspoon of pure vanilla extract

## Instructions

1. Mix all the ingredients for oatmeal except the vanilla in a medium saucepan. Stir to mix. The mixture should be brought to a boil over medium heat. Reduce heat to medium. Cook covered for 7 to 9 mins, occasionally stirring until the mixture thickens.
2. Stir in the vanilla. If desired, adjust the spices and sweetener.
3. Divide the oatmeal into bowls, and add your favorite toppings. The remaining leftovers can be kept in the refrigerator for up to five days in an airtight container. Reheat leftovers by adding them to a small saucepan with some coconut milk. Heat on medium heat until the mixture is well mixed. You can also enjoy cold leftovers!

# Faced Broiled Egg Spinach Tomato Sandwich

Prep time: 5 minutes

Cook time: 5 minutes

Serving: 1

## Ingredients

- 1/2 whole wheat English muffin
- 1/4 cup of fresh spinach cooked and squeezed dry
- 1 slice tomato
- 1 hard-boiled egg sliced widthwise
- 1 tablespoon of mayonnaise

## Instructions

1. Place half of the muffins on a baking sheet. Add tomato and spinach. Place egg slices in an overlaid spiral. Spread mayonnaise on egg slices and swirl it around to cover. Season with salt and pepper as needed
2. Broil for 2-3 minutes or until mayo is lightly browned.

# Omelette with Spinach and Tomato

Prep time: 5 minutes

Cook time: 5 minutes

Serving: 1

## Ingredients

- 2 teaspoons of olive oil
- 1 large vine tomato
- 2 handfuls of fresh spinach
- 2 eggs
- a splash of milk
- 20g Parmesan cheese
- sea salt and black pepper to season

## Instructions

1.  Heat a little oil or butter in a large frying pan and fry the spinach and tomato.
2.  Mix the eggs, milk and grated Parmesan. Season with salt and pepper.
3.  Turn the heat up to high.
4.  Place the eggs on top of the tomato and spinach. Stir the pan gently to coat everything.
5.  To cook the top of the Omelet, place the pan on a hot grill.

# Tropical Raspberry Smoothie

Prep time: 5 minutes

Cook time: 0 minutes

Serving: 1

## Ingredients

-   1/2 cup of frozen raspberries
-   1/2 cup of frozen pineapple chunks
-   1 banana, fresh
-   1 cup of orange-pineapple juice

## Introduction

1.  Blend the banana, orange pineapple juice, frozen pineapple chunks, frozen raspberries and frozen raspberries in a blender. Add yogurt if you're adding it. If the banana is fresh, it's not necessary to chop it up. You may need to cut the banana in half if frozen. If you freeze bananas yourself, it is a good idea to freeze them in chunks.
2.  Blend the juice and fruit on high for about a minute. Ensure the lid is securely secured to your blender to avoid an explosion. To create a smooth texture, reduce the speed of your blender to a lower setting.
3.  To enjoy the smoothie, pour it into a glass or container that can be used for storage. This smoothie can be shared with another person, but you can only drink it once.

# Roasted Vegetable Wrap with Feta and Pesto

Prep time: 10 minutes

Cook time: 20 minutes

Serving: 1

## Ingredients

- mixed vegetables cut into thin strips
- 1 teaspoon of olive oil
- salt and pepper, as needed
- 1 Flatout ProteinUp Carb Down wrap
- 1 tablespoon of prepared pesto
- 1 tablespoon of mayonnaise
- 1 tablespoon of crumbled feta cheese
- A handful of fresh baby spinach

## Instructions

1. Preheat oven to 425°F Place vegetables on a small sheet pan. Add olive oil, salt, and pepper. Bake for 10 minutes, then stir and roast until tender, approximately 10 minutes.
2. Mix pesto and mayonnaise in a small bowl until well-mixed. Spread the pesto evenly on Flatout Protein Up Carb Down wrap. Leave a 1-inch border around the wrap's edges.
3. Place roasted vegetables in the middle of the wrap. Top with feta cheese and spinach. Cover tightly. Enjoy immediately.

# Honey Lime Glazed Shrimp

Prep time: 1 minute

Cook time: 5 minutes

Serving: 4

## Ingredients

- ¼ cup of extra virgin olive oil
- 2 tablespoons of honey
- 2 limes juiced
- 2 teaspoons of minced garlic
- ¼ teaspoon of salt
- ¼ teaspoon of freshly cracked black pepper
- ½ teaspoon of chili powder
- ¼ teaspoon of paprika
- 1 lb shrimp peeled and deveined
- 2 tablespoons of fresh parsley chopped

## Instructions

1. Mix olive oil, honey lime juice, minced garlic and salt in a large bowl. Mix all ingredients. Whisk together.
2. Toss the shrimp in the marinade.
3. Marinate for at most 15 minutes to up to 8 hours
4. Over medium heat, heat the skillet. Add shrimp to the skillet and mix in the marinade.
5. Flip the shrimp after approximately 2 minutes.
6. Cook for 2-3 minutes until the shrimp become pink and curled.

# Chia, Hemp Hearts & Yogurt

Prep time: 2 minutes

Total time: 2 minutes

Serving: 1

## Ingredients

- 1 cup of Greek yogurt
- 1 tablespoon of chia seeds
- 1 tablespoon of hemp hearts
- 1 oz raspberries A handsful of raspberries
- 1 oz blackberries
- 1 oz walnuts

## Instructions

1. Make a yogurt breakfast bowl.
2. Blend in the berries, walnuts, then hemp hearts and chia seed.
3. Mix it all up and enjoy. If you prefer the flavor to be sweeter, add honey or vanilla greek. These options will give you sweeter tastes. Softened bananas can be added to the mix to sweeten the flavor.

# Matcha Chia Pudding

Prep time: 5 minutes

Cook time: 0 minutes

Serving: 2

## Ingredients

- 2 teaspoons of matcha green tea powder
- 1 cup of non-dairy milk
- ¼ cup of chia seeds
- ½ tablespoon of maple syrup
- Raspberries and almonds

## Instructions

1. Mix the matcha green tea powder and milk in a large bowl. Whisk until smooth.
2. Mix the maple syrup and chia seeds. Mix well, making sure that there are no lumps. Set it in the refrigerator for at least 2 hours.

# Apple Cinnamon Oatmeal Porridge

Prep time: 5 minutes

Cook time: 15 minutes

Serving: 2

## Ingredients

*OATMEAL:*

- 1 cup of thick-cut Rolled oats
- 1 medium Granny smith apple
- 4 cups of Almond milk
- ½ cup of condensed milk
- ¼ cup of pure maple syrup
- 1 tablespoon of ground cinnamon
- 1 teaspoon of ground nutmeg
- ½ teaspoon of ground allspice
- Pinch of sea salt

### CARAMELIZED APPLES:

- 1 medium Gala apples
- 2 Tablespoon of unsalted butter
- ½ cup of organic brown sugar
- 1 teaspoon of ground cinnamon
- pinch of sea salt

## Instructions

### To Make Oatmeal:

1. Mix the milk, oats and diced apples in a medium saucepan on medium heat. Stir until all is well mixed. Bring to a boil. Reduce heat to low and simmer for 8-10 minutes, stirring occasionally.
2. Once the oats are done, they should thicken and become swollen and fluffy, with half of the liquid remaining. Mix in the condensed milk and maple syrup. Let it simmer for another 1-2 minutes before you take it off the heat.

### Caramelized apples:

1. Heat the butter in a large skillet on medium heat. Stir in the brown sugar, cinnamon, and sea salt. Continue stirring until everything bubbles a little, approximately 2-3 minutes.
2. Toss the chopped apples with the sauce. Cook for 8-10 minutes until the apples are tender. Turn off the heat.
3. Serve oatmeal in a bowl. Top with caramelized apples, toasted nuts and maple syrup if you wish.

# Easy Overnight Oats

Prep time: 5 minutes

Total time: 5 minutes

Serving: 1

## Ingredients

### *Base*

- ½ cup of rolled oats
- ½ cup of milk of choice
- ¼ cup of non-fat Greek yogurt
- 1 tablespoon of chia seeds
- 1 tablespoon of sweetener honey or maple syrup
- ¼ teaspoon of vanilla extract

### *Peanut Butter & Jelly*

- 1 tablespoon of strawberry jam
- 1 tablespoon of creamy peanut butter
- ¼ cup of diced strawberries
- 2 tablespoons of peanuts crushed

### *Apple Pie*

- ¼ cup of diced apples
- 1 tablespoon of chopped pecans
- 2 teaspoons of maple syrup
- ¼ teaspoon of cinnamon

### *Banana Nutella*

- ½ banana sliced
- 1 tablespoon of Nutella
- 1 tablespoon of hazelnuts crushed
- 1 tablespoon of chocolate chips

### *Almond Joy*

- ¼ cup of shredded coconut
- 1 tablespoon of chopped almonds

- 1 tablespoon of chocolate chips
- 2 teaspoons of maple syrup

## Instructions

1. Mix all ingredients in a large container.
2. Use plastic wrap or a lid to cover the glass container. Place the container in the refrigerator for at most 2 hours. You can add toppings the night before or right before you serve.
3. Cover the container and let it sit for a day. If desired, thin it with some milk or water.

# Quinoa porridge

Prep time: 10 minutes

Cook time: 25 minutes

Serving: 4

## Ingredients

- For the porridge
- 175g quinoa
- ½ vanilla pod split, and seeds scraped
- 15g creamed coconut
- 4 tablespoons of chia seeds
- 125g coconut yogurt

## Instructions

1. Let the quinoa soak overnight in cold water to activate it. Drain the quinoa and rinse it with cold water.
2. In a saucepan, heat the quinoa. Add the vanilla, creamed coconut, and 600ml water. Let the mixture simmer on low heat for 20 minutes. Mix in the chia and 300ml of water. Continue to cook for 3 minutes. Add the coconut yogurt. Pour half of the porridge into a bowl and serve. Keeps for two days in the refrigerator. If you wish, serve the porridge with yogurt, berries, and almonds.
3. You can reheat the porridge with milk or water if you prefer it another day. Add fruit, such as orange slices or pomegranate seeds, to the porridge.

# Avocado & black bean eggs

Prep time: 5 minutes

Cook time: 5 minutes

Serving: 2

## Ingredients

- 2 teaspoons of rapeseed oil
- 1 red chili, deseeded and thinly sliced
- 1 large garlic clove, sliced
- 2 large eggs
- 400g can black beans
- ½ x 400g can cherry tomatoes
- ¼ teaspoon of cumin seeds
- 1 small avocado, halved and sliced
- a handful of fresh, chopped coriander
- 1 lime, cut into wedges

## Instructions

1. Heat the oil in a large nonstick frying pan. Stir in the chili and garlic, and cook until tender and beginning to turn golden. On each side, crack the eggs. Once the eggs start to set up, place the beans and tomatoes in a circle on the pan. Finally, sprinkle the cumin seeds. It is important to heat the beans and tomatoes, not to cook them.
2. Place the avocados and coriander in a pan and turn off the heat. Half of the lime wedges should be squeezed over. Serve with the remaining lime wedges on the side.

# Burger Bowl with Potato Hash

Prep time: 10 minutes

Cook time: 20 minutes

Serving: 4

## Ingredients

- 1 c diced russet potato
- 1 c diced sweet potato
- 1 strip bacon, diced
- 1/2 c diced onion
- 1/2 c diced bell pepper
- 1 Tablespoon of minced fresh parsley
- 1/2 Tablespoon of fresh thyme leaves, chopped
- 1/2 teaspoon of salt
- 1 lb lean ground beef
- salt as need
- pepper as need
- 1 avocado, diced
- 4 Davidson's Safest pasteurized egg
- chopped fresh parsley and thyme

## Instructions

1. Put potatoes in a microwave-safe bowl. Add 2 tablespoons of water. Cover the bowl with plastic wrap. Microwave on high for 2 minutes or until potatoes become partially cooked.
2. On medium heat, cook bacon in a large nonstick pan until the fat has rendered and the bacon is crisp. Cook and stir for one minute. Stir in bell pepper. Cook and stir for one more minute. Mix in the potatoes. Stir and scrape the pan from time to time until they are tender.
3. Add parsley, 1/2 teaspoon of salt, and thyme to the mixture. Spread the mixture evenly, pressing down lightly with a flat spatula. Allow the vegetables to brown for four minutes without stirring. Stir and spread the vegetables again. Cook for another 4 minutes, without stirring. Keep warm by covering the pan with a lid.
4. Season the beef patties on each side with salt & pepper: Grill pan or nonstick skillet on medium heat. Once patties are cooked, turn them over and continue cooking for about 5 minutes to achieve medium doneness (160degF).

5. Divide the hash between four bowls and sprinkle avocado on top. On each burger, place a sunny-side-down egg. Salt and pepper, fresh Parsley, and Thyme are some of the toppings for each egg.

# Banana Oat Pancakes

Prep time: 5 minutes

Cook time: 15 minutes

Serving: 2

## Ingredients

- 125ml oat milk
- 2 eggs, separated
- 1 small banana
- 100g rolled oats
- 2 teaspoons of baking powder
- few drops of vanilla extract
- oil
- low-fat yogurt and fruit to top

## Instructions

1. Blend the egg yolks and oat milk with the banana, oats and baking powder in a blender until you get a smooth mixture. Mix the egg whites with the sugar until they form stiff peaks. Mix 1-2 tablespoons of the whites in the batter and then fold it in.
2. Place a nonstick skillet on medium heat. Spray the pan with oil. Pour about 2 tablespoons of batter into the pan. Cook for approximately 1-2 minutes or until the batter is set and bubbles are visible. Flip the pancake and cook for one minute. You can do this in several batches. Make sure that the top is dry before you attempt the flip. Otherwise, the center may collapse.

# Farmers Market Breakfast Bow

Prep time: 20 minutes

Cook time: 10 minutes

Serving: 2

## Ingredients

- Spiced "Riced" Carrots:
- 2 medium carrots
- 2 teaspoons of lemon juice
- 1 teaspoon of extra-virgin olive oil
- ¼ teaspoon of cumin
- ¼ teaspoon of coriander
- sea salt and freshly ground black pepper

### *Yogurt Green Goddess Sauce*

- 2 cups of whole milk greek yogurt
- 2 tablespoons of lemon juice
- 2 tablespoons of extra-virgin olive oil
- 2 garlic cloves
- ½ teaspoon of sea salt
- ⅓ cup of chives, reserve
- ⅓ cup of fresh basil
- ¼ cup of fresh mint
- freshly ground black pepper

### *For the bowls:*

- a handful of salad greens
- 1 medium beet, shredded
- 4 radishes, thinly sliced
- 2 small tomatoes, sliced into wedges
- 2 soft-boiled eggs
- extra-virgin olive oil for drizzling
- sea salt and freshly ground black pepper

## Instructions

1. Make spiced carrot salad by grating the carrots. Toss the carrots in a bowl with olive oil, lemon juice, cumin, coriander, salt, and pinches more salt. Put the carrots aside.
2. Make the yogurt green goddess recipe: Use the Kitchen Aid 7 Cup of Food processor to puree the yogurt, lemon juice and olive oil until smooth. Blend in the mint, basil, chives and olive oil until well mixed.
3. Assemble the bowls by adding the greens, tomatoes, shredded beets, radishes and soft-boiled eggs. Season the bowls with olive oils and salt. Serve with a few spoonfuls of the yogurt sauce.
4. Keep the yogurt sauce refrigerated for up to four days. You can use it to dip vegetables, spread on sandwiches, or drizzle onto salads.

# Poached Eggs with Smashed Avocado & Tomatoes

Prep time: 10 minutes

Cook time: 10 minutes

Serving: 2

## Ingredients

- 2 tomatoes, halved
- ½ teaspoon of rapeseed oil
- 2 eggs
- 1 small ripe avocado
- 2 slices seeded wholemeal soda bread
- 2 handfuls rocket

## Instructions

1. Place the tomatoes in a nonstick frying pan. Lightly oil the tomatoes and then place them cut-side down in the pan. Cook until softened and lightly caramelized. In the meantime, heat some water. Once the eggs are boiled, add the eggs to the pan and let them cook for approximately 1-2 minutes.
2. Peel and slice the avocado. Then, scoop out the flesh and place it on the bread. Add the eggs to each bowl, and grind some black pepper. Serve the tomatoes alongside.

# Cinnamon Quinoa Breakfast Bowl

Prep time: 5 minutes

Cook time: 20 minutes

Serving: 2

## Ingredients

- ½ cup of uncooked quinoa
- 1 cup of Almond Breeze Almond milk
- 1-2 cinnamon sticks
- piece of a vanilla bean
- pinch of salt

### *Toppings:*

- toasted sliced almonds
- toasted coconut flakes
- peaches
- raspberries
- maple syrup, optional
- extra splashes of almond milk optional
- more spices, as need

## Instructions

1. Rinse the quinoa and drain it.
2. Add the almond milk, vanilla, cinnamon sticks, and salt to the saucepan. Cover and bring to a boil. Let it simmer for 15 minutes.
3. After 15 minutes, take the pan off the heat. Let the quinoa cool for five minutes or until the almond milk has been absorbed. Add additional spices to your taste.
4. Toss the quinoa into two bowls. Top with toasted almonds, coconut and other fruits. Maple syrup can be added if desired. You can serve it as a fluffy pilaf or as porridge with warm almond milk poured on top.

# Lentil Vegetable Soup

Prep time: 20 minutes

Cook time: 1 hour 30 minutes

Serving: 10

## Ingredients

- 1 lb. French green lentils
- 4 cups of chopped yellow onions
- 4 cups of chopped leeks, white part
- 1 tablespoon of minced garlic
- 1/4 cup of good olive oil
- 1 tablespoon of kosher salt
- 1 1/2 teaspoons of freshly ground black pepper
- 1 tablespoon of minced fresh thyme leaves
- 1 teaspoon of ground cumin
- 3 cups of medium diced celery
- 3 cups of medium diced carrot
- 3 quarts chicken stock
- 1/4 cup of tomato paste
- 2 tablespoons of red wine
- Freshly grated Parmesan cheese

## Instructions

1. Let the lentils 15 minutes to soak in a big dish of boiling water. Drain.
2. For 20 minutes, or until the veggies are translucent and very soft, sauté the onions, leeks, and garlic in the olive oil, salt, pepper, thyme, and cumin in a large stockpot over medium heat. Add the celery and carrots for ten more minutes and continue to sauté. Lentils, tomato paste, and chicken stock should all be added. Cover and heat until boiling. Lower the heat, cover the pot and simmer the lentils for an hour. Look through the seasonings. Red wine should be added before serving. Olive oil and grated Parmesan could also be added.

# Wild salmon veggie bowl

Prep time: 10 minutes

Cook time: 0 minutes

Serving: 2

## Ingredients

- 2 carrots
- 1large courgette
- 2 cooked beetroot, diced
- 2 tablespoons of balsamic vinegar
- ⅓ small pack of dill, chopped
- 1 small red onion, finely chopped
- 280g poached or canned wild salmon
- 2 tablespoons of capers in vinegar, rinsed

## Instructions

1. With a julienne peeler or spiralizer, shred the carrots and courgette into lengths like long spaghetti, then arrange them on two plates.
2. Mix the red onion, dill, balsamic vinegar, and beetroot; then, spread the mixture over the vegetables. Add chunks of flaked salmon and more dill, if desired, along with the capers.

# Sesame Soba Noodles

Prep time: 10 minutes

Cook time: 10 minutes

Serving: 6

## Ingredients

- 10 oz. HemisFares Soba Air-Dried Buckwheat Noodles
- ⅓ cup of HemisFares Double Fermented Soy Sauce
- 2 tablespoons of rice vinegar
- 3 tablespoons of toasted sesame oil
- ¼ teaspoon of freshly ground black pepper
- 1 tablespoon of sugar
- 1 tablespoon of canola oil
- 2 cups of green onions
- ½ cup of green onions
- 3 tablespoons of toasted sesame seeds

## Instructions

1. Soba noodles should be cooked for 4-5 minutes, or until just soft, in a big pot of boiling water, occasionally turning to prevent the noodles from sticking together. Drain in a strainer, then thoroughly rinse with cold water while tossing to get rid of the starch.
2. Mix the soy sauce, sesame oil, rice vinegar, sugar, and black pepper in a medium bowl while the noodles are boiling. Set aside.
3. Heat a large skillet over medium-high heat. Green onions that have been diced are added once the canola oil has shimmered. Sauté for 15 to 30 seconds while stirring until aromatic.
4. Cook the soy and sesame mixture for 30 seconds after adding. When the noodles are fully warm, add them and stir. Include the remaining green onion, minced, and half the sesame seeds. Serve hot or at room temperature and garnish with the remaining seeds.

# Lemon Zucchini Pasta Sauce with Feta

Prep time: 5 minutes

Cook time: 15 minutes

Serving: 1

## Ingredients

- 1 teaspoon of Olive Oil
- 1 medium Zucchini
- 2 teaspoons of lemon juice
- 60 g Short Pasta
- 50 g Feta Cheese
- Salt and Cracked Black Pepper as needed

## Instructions

1. Put a sizable pan of water on the stove to come to a boil; after it does, season it and cook your pasta as directed on the package.
2. Wash your zucchini, cut off the top and bottom, and chop it into bite-sized pieces. Keep the zucchini bite-sized; avoid cutting it into pieces larger than the pasta, as you want the lemon zucchini pasta sauce to mix nicely with the pasta.
3. Warm up the olive oil in a frying pan. When it's heated, stir in the zucchini and mix thoroughly.
4. The zucchini will be cooked in 8 to 10 minutes if you let them brown on a medium-low burner.
5. Dress the zucchini with half the lemon juice after they are finished cooking.
6. Drain the pasta from the water once it is finished cooking, and add it to the pan with the zucchini. Add salt, pepper, and lemon juice to dress it.
7. Add the crumbled feta right before serving, mix well, and plate. Enjoy!

# Poached Eggs with Broccoli, Tomatoes & Whole meal Flatbread

Prep time: 5 minutes

Cook time: 6 minutes

Serving: 2

## Ingredients

- 100g thin-stemmed broccoli, trimmed and halved
- 200g cherry tomatoes on the vine
- 4 medium free-range eggs
- 2 wholemeal flatbreads
- 2 teaspoons of mixed seeds

## Instructions

1. Burn the kettle. A heat-resistant plate should be placed into a 120°C oven to warm up. Bring to a boil a wide-based saucepan with a third of the water from the kettle filled with it. After adding, boil the broccoli for 2 minutes. 30 seconds after adding the tomatoes, bring the mixture back to a boil. When you poach the eggs, take them out with tongs or a slotted spoon and lay them on the heating dish in the oven.
2. Bring the water back to a low simmer. One at a time, crack the eggs into the pan and cook for two and a half to three minutes, or until the whites are set, and the yolks are still runny.
3. Place the tomatoes and broccoli on top of the flatbreads you have divided across the two plates. Place the eggs on top after draining with a slotted spoon. Add the seeds and the oil, then sprinkle. Serve right after adding some black pepper and red pepper flakes.

# Quinoa Stuffed Eggplant with Tahini Sauce

Prep time: 5 minutes

Cook time: 30 minutes

Serving: 2

## Ingredients

- 1 eggplant
- 2 tablespoons of olive oil divided
- 1 medium shallot diced
- 1 cup of chopped button mushrooms
- 6 Tuttorosso whole plum tomatoes chopped
- 1 tablespoon of tomato juice
- 2 garlic cloves minced
- 1/2 cup of cooked quinoa
- 1/2 teaspoon of ground cumin
- 1 tablespoon of chopped fresh parsley
- Salt & pepper as needed
- 1 tablespoon of tahini
- 1 teaspoon of lemon juice
- 1/2 teaspoon of garlic powder
- Water to thin

## Instructions

1. Set the oven's temperature to 425°F. Slice the eggplant lengthwise, then remove a portion of the flesh. Put in a baking sheet and cover with a thin layer of oil. Salt the top, then bake for 20 minutes.
2. Heat the remaining oil in a big pan while the eggplant cooks. Add the mushrooms and shallots all at once. Around 5 minutes of sautéing the mushrooms should soften them. Cook until the liquid has evaporated before including the tomatoes, quinoa, and seasonings.
3. Reduce the oven's heat to 350°F and fill each half of the eggplant with the tomato-quinoa mixture after it has cooked for 20 minutes. 10 more minutes of baking.
4. When ready to serve, mix tahini, water, lemon, garlic, and a little salt and pepper in a bowl. Tahini should be drizzled over the eggplants, then parsley should be added.

# Winter Veggie Power Bowl

Prep time: 10 minutes

Total time: 50 minutes

Serving: 2

## Ingredients

### Veggie Power Bowl

- 2 tablespoons of avocado oil
- 3 cups of cubed butternut squash
- 3 medium parsnips, peeled and cubed
- 1 teaspoon of garlic powder
- 1 large beet, peeled and cubed
- 1/2 teaspoon of cumin
- 6 cups of packed kale, roughly chopped
- 1/3 cup of walnuts
- 1/3 cup of dried cranberries
- 1 small avocado, sliced
- salt and pepper, as needed
- quinoa, chickpeas

### Vegan Tahini Dressing

- 2 tablespoons of tahini
- 2 tablespoons of coconut aminos
- 1 tablespoon of lemon juice
- 1 teaspoon of apple cider vinegar
- 1/4 teaspoon of ground ginger
- 1/4 teaspoon of garlic powder
- 1/4-1/2 teaspoon of red pepper flakes
- salt and pepper, as needed

## Instructions

1. The oven should be preheated to 375 degrees. 1–2 big baking sheets should be lined with parchment paper.
2. Vegetable roasting Butternut squash, partnerships, 1 tablespoon of avocado oil, garlic powder, salt, and pepper should all be mixed in a medium bowl. Put on a baking sheet, distributing vegetables evenly. Beets, 1/2 tablespoon of avocado

oil, cumin, salt, and pepper should all be added to the same bowl and mixed. If extra space is required, put it on the identical baking sheet or a different one. Roast for 35 to 40 minutes or until tender and soft.

3. Place the kale in a bowl and massage with 1/2 teaspoon of avocado oil, a sprinkle of salt, and pepper until the leaves are soft and pliable while the veggies roast.

4. Construct the dressing. All components are mixed in a bowl while being whisked. If you like a thinner or thicker consistency, respectively, add more water or more tahini.

5. Assemble the dishes after the vegetables are done. In three bowls, distribute the kale, roasted vegetables, walnuts, cranberries, and avocado. Add dressing over the top, then indulge!

# Warm Puttanesca Pasta Salad

Prep time: 10 minutes

Total time: 30 minutes

Serving: 4

## Ingredients

- 1 lb. cherry tomatoes, halved
- 1 teaspoon of kosher salt
- 1/2 teaspoon of freshly ground black pepper
- 1/4 cup of minced shallot
- 1/4 cup of extra-virgin olive oil
- 2 tablespoons of red wine vinegar
- 1 large garlic clove, grated
- 12 oz. uncooked casarecce pasta
- 4 prosciutto slices
- 3 oil-packed anchovies, finely chopped
- 1/2 cup of thinly sliced fresh basil
- 1/2 cup of coarsely chopped Castelvetrano olives
- 2 tablespoons of chopped fresh oregano
- 2 tablespoons of drained nonpareil capers
- Fresh basil leaves for garnish
- 1/2 teaspoon of cracked black pepper for garnish

## Instructions

1. Toss the tomatoes with salt and freshly ground pepper after placing them in a medium basin. Toss thoroughly after adding the shallot, oil, vinegar, and garlic. Let it rest for at least 20 minutes at room temperature.
2. Meanwhile, prepare pasta by following the directions on the box in salted water. Drain the pasta, saving 1 cup of the cooking water.
3. Put 2 slices of prosciutto on paper towels and place the plate in the microwave. 1 minute, 30 seconds to 2 minutes on HIGH, until crisp. Repeat with the remaining two pieces of prosciutto.
4. Over a basin, pour the tomato mixture and save the liquid. Mix the heated pasta, anchovies, tomato juice, and 1/3 cup of cooking liquid in a sizable skillet over medium-high heat over medium heat. Simmer for about 2 minutes until the sauce slightly thickens and coats the pasta. Get rid of the heat. Add the drained tomato mixture with the capers, olives, oregano, and basil slices. Pasta should be topped with crumbled prosciutto, basil, and, if preferred, cracked pepper.

# Greek-style roast fish

Prep time: 10 minutes

Cook time: 50 minutes

Serving: 2

## Ingredients

- 5 small potatoes, scrubbed
- 1 onion, halved and sliced
- 2 garlic cloves, roughly chopped
- ½ teaspoon of dried oregano
- 2 tablespoons of olive oil
- ½ lemon, cut into wedges
- 2 large tomatoes, cut into wedges
- 2 fresh skinless pollock fillets
- small handful parsley

## Instructions

1. Preheat oven to 200°C. Mix the potatoes, onion, garlic, oregano, salt, and pepper in a roasting pan. Next, stir everything with your hands to evenly distribute the oil. Turn everything over, and roast for a further 15 minutes.
2. The fish fillets should be added after the lemon and tomatoes have roasted for 10 minutes. Sprinkle parsley on top before serving.

# Baked Falafel Bowls

Prep time: 20 minutes

Cook time: 40 minutes

Serving: 4

## Ingredients

### For the Falafel:

- 2 cups of cooked chickpeas
- 1 cup of chopped parsley
- 3 large cloves of garlic
- 1 large lemon, juiced
- 1/2 teaspoon of sea salt
- 1 1/4 teaspoon of cumin
- 1/3 cup of almond meal

### For the Bowls:

- 1 cup of dry quinoa, cooked
- 1 large sweet potato, cubed
- 1 head of cauliflower, cut into florets
- 2 tablespoons of olive oil
- sea salt

### For the Tahini Dressing:

- 4 tablespoons of tahini
- 1 lemon, juiced
- 2–4 tablespoons of water
- 1 garlic clove, minced
- 1 tablespoon of za'atar

## Instructions

### *For the Falafels:*

1. Preheat oven to 400°F and line a baking sheet using parchment or a silicone pad.
2. Add all ingredients to a food processor except for an almond meal.
3. Pulse the mixture until it is fully mixed, scraping any sides as necessary.
4. Add an almond meal. The mixture should retain its shape if it doesn't, add almond meal as necessary.
5. Take 2 tablespoons of the mixture and form a ball.
6. Bake for 10 minutes, then flip and bake for another 10 minutes.

### *For the Bowls:*

1. Place sweet potato and cauliflower on a baking sheet. Drizzle olive oil over the top.
2. Sprinkle with sea salt, and bake for between 30-40 minutes.
3. Serve cooked quinoa, sweet potato, and cauliflower bowls with falafel.

### *For the Dressing:*

1. Mix all ingredients together and add water to achieve desired consistency.
2. Serve in bowls.

# Baked Eggs with Tomatoes and Feta Cheese

Prep time: 5 minutes

Cook time: 15 minutes

Serving: 2

## Ingredients

- 1/2 cup of Beefsteak tomato, chopped
- 1/2 cup of Feta Cheese, good quality, crumbled
- 4 eggs
- 1/4 teaspoon of dried oregano
- Olive Oil Spray

## Instructions

1. Preheat the oven to 350 F

2. Olive oil spray can be used to spray ramekins
3. To ramekins, add chopped tomatoes and crumbled feta.
4. Sprinkle with dried oregano
5. Add 2 eggs to each ramekin.
6. Sprinkle with freshly grated pepper and salt.
7. Bake it for about 15-17 minutes.

# Egg Nicosia salad

Prep time: 10 minutes

Cook time: 10 minutes

Serving: 2

## Ingredients

### For the dressing

- 2 tablespoons of rapeseed oil
- juice 1 lemon
- 1 teaspoon of balsamic vinegar
- 1 garlic clove, grated
- ⅓ small pack of basil leaves chopped
- 3 pitted black Kalamata olive

### For the salad

- 2 eggs
- 250g new potatoes, thickly sliced
- 200g fine green beans
- ½ red onion, very finely chopped
- 14 cherry tomatoes, halved
- 6 romaine lettuce leaves
- 6 pitted black Kalamata olive

## Instructions

1. Mix the dressing ingredients in a small bowl. Add 1 tablespoon of water.
2. Boil the potatoes for 7 minutes, then add the beans. Cook the beans for 5 minutes more or until they are tender. Drain the excess water. Boil 2 eggs for 8 mins, then shell and halves.

3. Mix the beans, potatoes, and other salad ingredients except for the eggs in a large bowl. Add half of the dressing to the bowl. Place the eggs on top of the dressing and drizzle the rest over.

# Cucumber Sandwiches

Prep time: 20 minutes

Total time: 20 minutes

Serving: 32

## Ingredients

- 16 slices high-quality soft white sandwich bread, crusts removed
- 1 English cucumber
- 8 oz. cream cheese, softened
- 1/4 cup of mayonnaise
- 1 tablespoon of minced fresh dill
- 1 tablespoon of minced fresh chives
- 1 tablespoon of lemon juice
- 1/4 teaspoon of garlic powder
- 1/4 teaspoon of kosher salt
- Cracked black pepper, as need

## Instructions

1. Cut the cucumber into thin strips into 1/8-inch slices using a mandolin. Sprinkle coarse salt on the slices and place them on paper towels. Allow resting for between 15 and 30 minutes to draw out moisture. Use clean paper towels to dry.
2. Make the spread while you wait. Blend the softened cream cheese with mayo, dill and chives in a large bowl. Add the garlic powder, lemon juice, garlic powder, salt, and pepper.
3. Place the herbed cream cheese on one side of each bread slice.
4. Layer cucumber slices on half the bread slices. Season with freshly cracked black pepper as needed. Add the remaining bread slices and cream cheese mixture to the top.
5. Use a sharp chef's knife to cut each sandwich into quarters. Push the bread through the bottom. You now have 32 tea sandwiches.
6. Serve immediately and enjoy.

# BLT Pasta Salad

Prep time: 25 minutes

Total time: 25 minutes

Serving: 10

## Ingredients

- 1 12-oz. package bacon
- 1 16-oz. box of fusilli or curly pasta
- 1 c. mayonnaise
- 3/4 c. whole milk
- 1 1-oz. packet ranch seasoning mix
- Juice of one lemon
- 1/4 c. grated parmesan cheese
- 1/2 teaspoon of ground black pepper
- 1-pint grape tomatoes halved
- 2 c. thinly sliced romaine lettuce
- 1/2 c. chopped red onion
- 1/4 c. chopped fresh herbs

## Instructions

1. In a large pan over medium heat, cook the bacon, flipping as necessary, for 8 to 10 minutes, or until the fat has rendered and the bacon is golden and crispy. Crumble the bacon into bite-sized pieces after it cools to room temperature.
2. The pasta should be prepared as directed on the packaging. Drain, give a cold water rinse, and let it cool.
3. In a large bowl, mix the mayonnaise, milk, ranch seasoning, lemon juice, parmesan cheese, and black pepper. Add pasta, tomatoes, lettuce, onion, herbs, and half of the crumbled bacon to the dressing-filled dish. Coat by gently folding them together. Serve with the leftover bacon on top.

# Stovetop Turmeric Oatmeal

Prep time: 5 minutes

Total time: 5 minutes

Serving: 2

## Ingredients

- 1 mashed banana
- 1.5 cups of oats
- 2 cups of milk of choice
- 3/4 teaspoon of ground turmeric
- ¼ salt
- ¼ teaspoon of ground ginger
- ¼ teaspoon of cinnamon
- 1 Tablespoon of maple syrup
- 1 Tablespoon of chia seeds
- pinch of black pepper, optional

## Instructions

1. Use a fork to mash your banana in a bowl.
2. Mix your oats, milk, turmeric, salt, ginger, cinnamon, and maple syrup in a small or medium pot.
3. Chia seeds are added to boiling oats, which are then simmered for three to five minutes to thicken.
4. Serve with your preferred garnishes!

# Chicken Casserole

Prep time: 10 minutes

Cook time: 4 hours 15 minutes

Serving: 2

## Ingredients

- knob of butter
- ½ tablespoon of rapeseed or olive oil
- 1 large onion, finely chopped
- 1 ½ tablespoons of flour
- 650g boneless, skinless chicken thigh fillets
- 3 garlic cloves, crushed
- 400g baby new potatoes, halved
- 2 sticks celery, diced
- 2 carrots, diced
- 250g mushrooms, quartered
- 15g dried porcini mushroom
- 500ml chicken stock cubes
- 2 teaspoons of Dijon mustard
- 2 bay leaves

## Instructions

1. 1 big onion, finely diced, cooked in a large frying pan with a knob of butter and 1/2 tablespoon of rapeseed or olive oil for 8 to 10 minutes or until tender and beginning to caramelize.
2. Meanwhile, mix 650g boneless, skinless chicken thigh fillets with 1 1/2 tablespoons of flour, some salt, and pepper in a bowl.
3. Cook the chicken in the skillet with 3 smashed garlic cloves for another 4-5 minutes or until it begins to brown.
4. Add 400 grams of halved baby new potatoes, two diced celery sticks, two diced carrots, 250 grams of quartered mushrooms, 15 grams of dried and soaked porcini mushrooms with the 50 milliliter soaking liquid, 500 milliliters of chicken stock, two teaspoons of Dijon mustard, and two bay leaves to your slow cooker.
5. Stir it thoroughly. Cook for 7 hours on low or 4 hours on high.
6. Take off the bay leaves before serving, and add some Dijon mustard.

# Salmon Sandwich with Whipped Goat's Cheese

Prep time: 10 minutes

Cook time: 10 minutes

Serving: 2

## Ingredients

- 4 slices of bread of your choice
- 200 g smoked salmon
- 100 g soft goat's cheese
- 2 tablespoons of sour cream
- 1 tablespoon of chives finely chopped
- ½ red onion thinly sliced
- 2 tablespoons of microgreens
- 2 tablespoons of capers/caper berries.
- fresh lemon juice as needed
- salt and pepper as needed

## Instructions

1. Mix the goat cheese, sour cream, lemon juice, salt, and pepper in the bowl of a food processor. Once smooth, blend.
2. Toast the bread in a hot pan until golden brown for more texture.
3. The smoked salmon ribbons should be layered on top of a liberal amount of goat cheese.
4. Add capers, thin red onion slices, and microgreens on the top. Add some freshly squeezed lemon juice and a sprinkle of black pepper.
5. Serve right away.

# Blueberry Protein Pancakes

Prep time: 5 minutes

Total time: 15 minutes

Serving: 12

## Ingredients

- 1 1/2 cups of almond flour
- 1/2 cup of protein powder
- 1 1/2 teaspoons of baking powder
- 1/2 teaspoon of cinnamon
- 3 eggs
- ⅔ cup of almond milk
- 1/2 - 1 cup of blueberries

## Instructions

1. The dry ingredients should be thoroughly mixed and placed aside.
2. A dish of dry ingredients for protein pancakes.
3. The eggs and almond milk are mixed in a separate bowl. Add a dash of vanilla if you'd like a tiny flavor boost.
4. Bowl of wet ingredients for protein pancakes.
5. Stirring will be necessary after adding the egg and milk combination to the flour mixture. Blueberries are folded in.
6. The wet and dry components of a protein pancake are mixed in a bowl.
7. Spray cooking spray in a skillet that has been heated to medium-low heat. On each side, fry the batter for 2 to 3 minutes after dropping roughly a 1/4 cup of it onto the pan. Replicate with the remaining batter.
8. In a skillet, a protein pancake.
9. Warm pancakes should be served with vegan yogurt and real maple syrup.

# Grilled Turkey-Zucchini Burgers

Prep time: 10 minutes

Cook time: 25 minutes

Serving: 4

## Ingredients

- 1 medium zucchini, grated
- 1 lb. 85% lean ground turkey
- 1 large egg
- 1 teaspoon of garlic powder
- 1 teaspoon of ground cumin
- 50 teaspoons of kosher salt
- Canola oil for grilling
- 4 burger buns, toasted
- Sliced tomatoes, Bibb lettuce, mayonnaise, honey mustard, and pickles for topping
- Sweet potato chips for serving

## Instructions

1. Put the zucchini on a clean dish towel, then squeeze out any extra liquid. Mix the squeezed zucchini with the turkey, egg, garlic powder, cumin, and salt in a large bowl. Four equal pieces of the ingredients should be formed into patties that are each 34 inches thick.
2. An oiled grill or a greased grill pan should be heated to medium or medium-high. Add the patties and cook, turning once, for 5 to 6 minutes on each side or until a thermometer inserted in the middle of the patties reads 165 F. Serve with chosen toppings, chips, and buns.

# Tuna Melt Grilled Cheese Sandwich

Prep time: 5 minutes

Cook time: 5 minutes

Serving: 4

## Ingredients

- 2 cans Tuna, drained
- 1/4 cup of Mayonnaise
- 2 Tablespoon of Onion, finely diced
- 1 cup of Shredded Cheddar Cheese
- 8 slices White Bread
- Butter softened

## Instructions

1. Mix tuna, mayonnaise, and chopped onion in a small bowl. Add cheddar cheese and mix gently.
2. Each bread slice should have butter on one side.
3. Over medium heat, warm the skillet. Take one slice of bread and set it butter side down on the griddle to construct a sandwich. To the tuna mixture, add 1/4. Put onto bread slice. The second slice of bread should be placed on top, butter side up. Flip the bread over when the bottom has browned to brown the other side.
4. Add the remaining ingredients and repeat. Serve hot with pickles and chips on the side.

# Couscous & Pear Salad with Goat's Cheese

Prep time: 10 minutes

Cook time: 12 minutes

Serving: 2

## Ingredients

- ½ cup of couscous
- ½ cup of water + 2 tablespoon of
- ¼ teaspoon of salt
- 2 handful baby spinach or torn kale leaves
- 1 pear
- 3 oz goat cheese
- 1 tablespoon of maple syrup
- 1 tablespoon of balsamic vinegar
- ½ teaspoon of olive oil

## Instructions

1. Lightly roast the couscous in the oven for about 1-2 minutes until it turns light brown, and the aroma is released. Next, move on to step 2. You can skip this step to save time.
2. Place the couscous in a medium-sized bowl. Mix 1/2 cup of boiling water with 1/4 teaspoon of salt. Cover the bowl and let it sit for 8-10 minutes.
3. 1/2 cup of couscous, 1/2 Cup of water + 2 Tablespoon of Flaky or Sea Salt
4. Toss in baby spinach, torn kale leaves and sliced pear. Add goat cheese to the bowl. Add maple syrup, balsamic vinegar, olive oil, and 2 Tablespoon of water, and generously sprinkle with flaky salt or sea salt. Mix well and serve.
5. 2 handfuls of baby spinach, torn kale, 1 pear,3 oz goat cheddar,1 tablespoon of maple syrup, and 1 teaspoon of balsamic vinegar. Flaky sea salt, 1/2 teaspoon of olive oil

# Roast sea bass & vegetable traybake

Prep time: 10 minutes

Cook time: 30 minutes

Serving: 2

## Ingredients

- 300g red-skinned potatoes
- 1 red pepper, cut into strips
- 2 tablespoons of extra virgin olive oil
- 1 rosemary sprig, leaves removed
- 2 sea bass fillets
- 25g pitted black olive, halved
- ½ lemon, sliced thinly into rounds
- handful basil leaves

## Instructions

1. Preheat oven to 180C/160C fan/gas 4. Place the pepper and potato slices on a large, nonstick baking sheet. Sprinkle the oil with the rosemary and salt. Mix everything well. Roast for 25 minutes, turning once halfway through until potatoes are crisp around the edges.
2. Place the fish fillets on the top. Sprinkle the olives over them. Sprinkle the remaining oil over the fish. Continue roasting for another 7-8 minutes until the fish is fully cooked. Sprinkle with basil leaves.

# Mango Ginger Rice Bowl

Prep time: 20 minutes

Cook time: 5 minutes

Serving: 2

## Ingredients

- 2 handfuls snap peas, strings removed
- 1 to 2 cups of cooked short-grain white rice
- 2 cups of shredded green cabbage
- 1 small carrot, sliced into very thin coins
- ½ English cucumber
- 1 small ripe ataulfo mango
- ½ cup of cooked black beans
- 2 tablespoons of pickled ginger
- ¼ cup of thinly sliced fresh basil
- ¼ cup of toasted peanuts, optional
- A sprinkle of sesame seeds, optional
- ¼ to ½ avocado, optional

### *Dressing*

- 2 tablespoons of tamari
- 2 tablespoons of rice vinegar
- 2 tablespoons of lime juice
- 2 garlic cloves, minced
- 2 teaspoons of cane sugar
- ½ teaspoon of sriracha

## Instructions

1. Mix together the tamari and vinegar, lime juices, garlic, cane sugar, and Sriracha in a small bowl.
2. Bring a small saucepan of salted water over medium heat. Add a bowl of ice water to the pot. To blanch the snap peas, boil them for about 1 1/2 minutes. Then scoop them into the ice water to stop the cooking process. Drain the snap peas once they have cooled. Pat dry and chop.
3. The bowls should be filled with rice, shredded cabbage and carrots, as well as cucumbers, mangoes, black beans, pickled ginger, and basil. If desired, top the bowls with avocado, sesame seeds, and toasted peanuts. Serve half of the

dressing in bowls. If desired, add the remaining dressing to the bowl and garnish with tamari or sriracha.

# Orzo, bean and tuna salad

Prep time: 5 minutes

Total time: 20 minutes

Serving: 2

## Ingredients

- ½ red onion, finely chopped
- 2 tablespoons of sherry vinegar
- 150g green beans, cut
- 100g orzo
- 1 tablespoon of olive oil
- 1 tin tuna, drained and flaked
- 3 roasted red peppers from a jar
- 12 dry-cured black olives, halved
- a handful of dill, chopped

## Instructions

1. Place the onions, vinegar, and seasoning in a bowl.
2. After 3 minutes of boiling in salted water, remove the beans using a slotted spoon. Orzo should be cooked in the same water until just soft, then drained, rinsed with cold water, and thoroughly drained once more.
3. Pour the beans, orzo, olive oil, tuna, peppers, olives, dill, and salt and pepper as needed into the dish with the onion. Mix, then plate.

# Smoked Tofu and Hummus Buddha Bowl

Prep time: 5 minutes

Cook time: 10 minutes

Serving: 2

## Ingredients

- ½ teaspoon of turmeric
- ½ cup of basmati rice
- 10 oz smoked tofu
- 2 teaspoons of olive oil
- 2 handful lamb's lettuce
- 1 small red onion
- 6 tablespoons of hummus
- 1 tablespoon of lemon juice
- 8 tablespoons of water
- ½ teaspoon of salt

## Instructions

1. Rice should be prepared as directed on the box. Add salt and turmeric and stir. You should know that the rice-to-water ratio is 2:1. With a cover on top, simmer for 10 minutes with cold water that has been brought to a boil. Done
2. Slice the smoked tofu. Next, preheat a skillet over medium heat, add the olive oil, and add the tofu, cubed. It takes around 7 minutes to fry.
3. Slice the red onion thinly and clean the lamb's lettuce. Place both in your dish after that.
4. Hummus, lemon juice, and water are added to a small bowl. Be sure to mix thoroughly.
5. Put the cooked rice and fried tofu in your bowl to assemble. Pour the hummus dressing over it at this point. If necessary, season with salt.
6. Enjoy!

# Lighter Chinese chili beef

Prep time: 35 minutes

Cook time: 10 minutes

Serving: 2

## Ingredients

- 250g lean beef, such as sirloin steak
- ½ red pepper
- 4 spring onions, ends trimmed
- 85g Tenderstem broccoli spears
- 100g pak choi
- 3 tablespoons of fresh orange juice
- 1 teaspoon of Chinese rice wine vinegar
- 2 teaspoons of dark soy sauce
- 1 teaspoon of hot chili sauce, such as sriracha
- 1 medium egg white
- ½ teaspoon of five-spice powder
- 1 tablespoon of cornflour
- 1 ½ teaspoon of self-raising flour
- 1 tablespoon plus 1 ½ teaspoons of rapeseed oil
- 2 garlic cloves, finely chopped
- 2 teaspoons of finely chopped root ginger
- ¼ teaspoon of chili flakes

## Instructions

1. The meat should be frozen for between 25 and 30 minutes before you start cooking. This will help to firm the meat and make it easier for you to cut thinly.
2. Cut the pepper into thin strips by removing the seeds and core. Cut the spring onions into diagonal slices. Slice the broccoli spears in quarters or half through the stems. Slice the pakchoi thinly. Mix the orange juice vinegar, soy sauce, chili sauce, and soy sauce. Set aside.
3. Cut the beef into thin strips. Mix the egg white in a bowl until it is slightly foamy. Stir in the beef and the cornflour, flour, five-spice powder, and pepper. Make sure everything is well coated. Place 1 tablespoon of oil in a nonstick wok/frying pan. Once the oil is very hot (test it by dropping a piece of beef into it - it should immediately sizzle), add the beef and stir to separate. Continue cooking for about 3-4 minutes. Remove the beef with a slotted spoon.

4. The broccoli spears should be boiled for about 11/2 minutes. Next, place the pakchoi on top of the broccoli spears and steam them for 45 seconds to 1 minute until they are tender-crisp. Let cool in a bowl of cold water until they are no longer cooked. Set aside.

5. Heat the remaining oil in the wok until it is hot. Stir-fry the spring onions, garlic, ginger, red pepper, and red pepper for 2 minutes until they start to brown. The chili flakes can be added to the mixture. Next, add the orange juice and soy sauce along with about 4-5 tablespoons of water. Once the water has come to a boil, add the beef and steamed vegetables and stir. You can add another 2 to 3 tablespoons of water if you like it a bit saucier.

# Chipotle chicken lunch wrap

Prep time: 5 minutes

Total time: 35 minutes

Serving: 2

## Ingredients

- 2 small chicken breasts
- 2 tablespoons of chipotle paste
- ¼ red cabbage, shredded
- 2 spring onions, thinly sliced
- 1 lime, juiced
- 2 handfuls of baby spinach
- large handful of coriander, chopped
- 2 large tortilla wraps, wholemeal
- 2 tablespoons of soured cream
- 2 tablespoons of pickled jalapeños, chopped
- Tabasco, to serve

## Instructions

1. The oven should be heated to 200C/fan 180C/gas 6. Season the chicken breasts with the chipotle paste. Bake in the oven for 20-25 mins or until cooked through. Let cool on the tray for five minutes before slicing and then tossing with any juices.

2. Mix the cabbage and spring onion together, then season with lime juice. Use clean hands to massage the cabbage with spring onion. Next, add the spinach and coriander.
3. Spread the soured cream on a large foil sheet on a cutting board. Spread the soured cream a third of the way up each tortilla. Layer half the chicken horizontally on top. Top it with half of the slaw mixture. Finish the dish by adding jalapenos and Tabasco if desired. The foil can be used to fold the tortilla in half. Once the tortilla is folded in half, use it to roll the tortilla around itself. Continue with the rest of the ingredients and tortilla. Each tortilla can be cut in half for easy serving.

# Slow-Cooker Chicken Curry

Prep time: 10 minutes

Cook time: 6 hours

Serving: 2

## Ingredients

- 1 large onion, roughly chopped
- 3 tablespoons of mild curry paste
- 400g can of chopped tomatoes
- 2 teaspoons of vegetable bouillon powder
- 1 tablespoon of finely chopped ginger
- 1 yellow pepper, deseeded and chopped
- 2 skinless chicken legs, fat removed
- 30g pack fresh coriander, leaves chopped
- cooked brown rice to serve

## Instructions

1. Stir well after adding one large onion that has been roughly chopped, three tablespoons of mild curry paste, a can of chopped tomatoes that weighs 400 grams, two teaspoons of vegetable bouillon powder, one tablespoon of finely chopped ginger, and one tablespoon of yellow pepper to the slow cooker pot.
2. 2 skinless, fat-free chicken legs should be added and pushed beneath everything else, so they are totally immersed. Overnight in the refrigerator, cover with the lid.

3. Cook the chicken and veggies on Low for 6 hours the following day to make sure they are really soft.
4. Just before serving the brown rice over the 30g of chopped coriander, stir in the mixture.

# Kimchi Brown Rice Bliss Bowls

Prep time: 10 minutes

Cook time: 30 minutes

Serving: 2

## Ingredients

- 1 cup of cooked brown rice
- Heaping ¼ cup of kimchi
- 1 Persian cucumber, peeled into ribbons
- ½ cup of thinly sliced red cabbage
- ½ avocado, sliced
- 8 oz. Marinated Tempeh, Baked or Grilled
- ½ recipe Peanut Sauce
- ½ teaspoon of sesame seeds
- 2 Thai chiles, thinly sliced, optional
- Lime slices for serving
- Microgreens, for garnish, optional

## Instructions

1. Assemble the bowls by adding the rice, kimchi and cucumber to the bowls.
2. Sprinkle a generous amount of peanut sauce over the top. If desired, sprinkle sesame seeds or Thai chiles on top. Serve with lime slices, remaining peanut sauce and the rest of the peanut sauce. If desired, garnish with microgreens.

# Grilled Chicken Wrap

Prep time: 10 minutes

Cook time: 10 minutes

Serving: 2

## Ingredients

- 2 chicken breasts sliced into cutlets
- 1 teaspoon of smoked paprika
- ¼ teaspoon of chili powder
- ½ teaspoon of garlic granules
- ½ teaspoon of salt
- ⅛ teaspoon of ground black pepper
- 1 tablespoon of oil if frying
- 4 tortillas
- 4 large iceberg lettuce
- 1 cup of cheddar or mozzarella cheese shredded
- ½ cup of ranch dressing

## Instructions

1. Salt, pepper, chili powder, smoked paprika, garlic powder, and other seasonings are used to season the chicken cutlets.
2. Preheat your outside grill or a grill pan by heating the oil.
3. Cook the chicken cutlets on the grill or in a pan until it is well done on both sides. The chicken must have an internal temperature of at least 165°F (75°C) in the core.
4. The chicken should be taken off the grill and given five minutes to rest on a platter.
5. After chopping the chicken, put the wrap together.
6. To assemble, place lettuce leaves on tortilla bread, then add chicken, shredded cheese, and ranch dressing. Place the tortilla wrap on the grill after sealing it. Sauté the wraps for one or two minutes on each side, then remove, cut them in half, and serve.

# Green Goddess Cream Cheese Veggie Sandwich

Prep time: 15 minutes

Cook time: 6 minutes

Serving: 2

## Ingredients

- 7 oz. Light cream cheese
- 2 tablespoons of Italian flat-leaf parsley
- 2 tablespoons of basil leaves
- 1 tablespoon of tarragon leaves
- 1 ½ teaspoons of chives , minced
- 1 small garlic clove, pressed
- ¼ lemon, juiced
- kosher salt and freshly ground black pepper
- 4 slices thick-cut sandwich bread
- Extra virgin olive oil
- ½ zucchini, sliced
- Fresh baby spinach leaves
- thinly sliced Cucumber
- thickly sliced Heirloom green tomato
- pitted and sliced Avocado
- Broccoli or alfalfa sprouts

## Instructions

1. Mix the parsley, basil, tarragon, chives, garlic, and lemon juice with the cream cheese in a small bowl. Set aside after seasoning with freshly ground black pepper and kosher salt as needed.
2. A grill pan should be heated very hot. Salt and pepper the zucchini slices after brushing them with olive oil. After 3 minutes, turn the zucchini slices over and cook the other side as before. Take out of the pan and place somewhere to cool.
3. Each slice of bread should have the cream cheese mixture spread on one side.
4. Then, layer the following veggies over the cream cheese mixture on two pieces of bread: slices of zucchini, baby spinach, cucumber, tomato, and avocado. Top with sprouts after adding a dash of kosher salt and add freshly ground black pepper. Slice the top piece of bread in half and serve it over the sprouts. Any excess cream cheese should be saved for further use or more sandwiches.

# Ginger chicken & green bean noodles

Prep time: 10 minutes

Cook time: 15 minutes

Serving: 2

## Ingredients

- ½ tablespoon of vegetable oil
- 2 skinless chicken breasts, sliced
- 200g green beans, trimmed
- a thumb-sized piece of ginger, peeled
- 2 garlic cloves, sliced
- 1 ball stem ginger, finely sliced
- 1 teaspoon of cornflour
- 1 teaspoon of dark soy sauce,
- 2 teaspoons of rice vinegar
- 200g cooked egg noodles

## Instructions

1. The oil in a wok is heated over high heat while the chicken is stir-fried for 5 minutes. When the chicken is just cooked through, add the green beans and stir-fry for an additional 4-5 minutes.
2. Fresh ginger and garlic should be stir-fried for two minutes before stem ginger, syrup, cornflour mixture, soy sauce, and vinegar are added. After one minute of stirring, add the noodles. Cook the food until it's all hot and the sauce has coated the noodles. If desired, drizzle on extra soy before serving.

# Spicy Salmon Poke Bowls

Prep time: 25 minutes

Cook time: 5 minutes

Serving: 4

## Ingredients

### *Sockeye Salmon*

- 1 lb. sockeye salmon, cut
- ¼ cup of soy sauce, low sodium
- 1 teaspoon of rice wine vinegar
- 1 teaspoon of sriracha or chili paste
- 1 teaspoon of sesame oil

### *Pickled Cucumbers*

- 2 6-inch Persian cucumbers, thinly sliced
- ½ cup of rice wine vinegar, Kikkoman
- ½ cup of water
- ⅓ cup of honey
- 1 teaspoon of kosher salt
- ½ teaspoon of red chili flakes, dried

### *Sriracha Sauce*

- 2 tablespoons of sriracha
- 2 tablespoons of plain greek yogurt

## Instructions

1. Mix the chopped salmon, soy sauce, vinegar, sriracha, and sesame oil in a medium bowl. Add a cover and chill.
2. In a medium saucepan, mix the vinegar, water, honey, salt, and chili flakes. Over high heat, bring to a boil.
3. Once boiling, turn off the heat and mix in the cucumber slices.
4. After 10 minutes of resting, move the cucumber to a container, cover it, and store it in the refrigerator until needed.
5. Stir together 2 teaspoons of Sriracha and 2 tablespoons of yogurt or mayonnaise in a small dish.

6. When ready to serve, add any extra items to the bowl's foundation (such as rice or salad). Add other toppings, such as pickled cucumbers and 1/2 cup of salmon poke, on top. Pour on some Sriracha sauce.

# Lentil Bowls with Avocado, Eggs and Cholula

Prep time: 5 minutes

Total time: 5 minutes

Serving: 2

## Ingredients

- 1½cups of lentils, cooked
- squeeze of lime
- kosher salt and black pepper, as need
- 3 large hard-boiled eggs, peeled
- 2ozavocado,sliced
- ½cup of grape tomatoes halved
- cilantro, chopped
- Cholula hot sauce, a few dashes

## Instructions

1. Add 3 egg halves, 1 oz. of avocado, 1 tablespoon of cilantro, and extra salt and pepper to a bowl with 1/4 cup of lentils. Squeeze a little lime juice over the top and season with salt and pepper as needed.
2. Add spicy sauce to the end, then enjoy!

# Sweet & Sour Stir-Fry

Prep time: 5 minutes

Cook time: 21 minutes

Serving: 2

## Ingredients

- 100 g fine rice noodles
- 1 x 227 g tin of pineapple chunks in juice
- 2 heaped teaspoons of cornflour
- 1 tablespoon of cider vinegar
- 2 teaspoons of low-salt soy sauce
- 2 teaspoons of sesame seeds
- 30 g cashew nuts
- 4 spring onions
- 2 cloves of garlic
- 2 cm piece of ginger
- 1 fresh red chili
- 200 g sugar snap peas
- groundnut oil
- 200 g sprouts, such as alfalfa sprouts
- 1 lime

## Instructions

1. Pour boiling kettle water over 100g of fine rice noodles into a dish to rehydrate them.
2. The juice from one 227g can of pineapple chunks be drained into a separate bowl, where it should be mixed with 2 heaping teaspoons of cornflour, 1 tablespoon of cider vinegar, 2 teaspoons of low-salt soy sauce, and 4 tablespoons of water to make a sauce. This sauce should then be set aside.
3. 2 tablespoons of sesame seeds should be gently toasted in a wok or big frying pan over high heat before being poured into a small bowl.
4. After adding 30g of the coarsely chopped cashew nuts and waiting a few minutes, add the pineapple pieces to the dry pan.

5. 4 spring onions should be cleaned and then cut into slices of 2 cm. As you peel and thinly slice 200g of sugar snaps at an angle lengthways, 2 cloves of garlic, a 2 cm piece of ginger, and 1 fresh red chili, let everything brown and become moody.

6. Add the garlic, ginger, and chili to the pan, along with 1 tablespoon of groundnut oil. Stir for 30 seconds. Add the sugar snap peas and the more vigorous sprouts, stir for a further minute, then add the sauce. For a few minutes to thicken, bring it to a boil. After that, taste it and adjust the seasoning as needed.

7. Over the drained noodles, plate the stir-fry. Return the empty pan to the fire as soon as possible, add a generous amount of boiling kettle water, and use a wooden spoon to thoroughly scrape up all the yummy sticky deliciousness from the bottom. Stir for 1 minute, until the mixture has slightly thickened, then drizzle it over the stir-fry.

8. Serve with lime wedges on the side for squeezing over any delicate sprouts, such as alfalfa, and top with the toasted sesame seeds.

# Pasta with Salmon & Peas

Prep time: 5 minutes

Cook time: 10 minutes

Serving: 2

## Ingredients

- 240g wholewheat fusilli
- knob of butter
- 1 large shallot, finely chopped
- 140g frozen peas
- 2 skinless salmon fillets cut into chunks
- 140g low-fat crème fraîche
- ½ low-salt vegetable stock cube
- small bunch of chives snipped

## Instructions

1. Cook the fusilli per the directions on the package in a pan of boiling water.
2. Meanwhile, soften the shallot by cooking it in a pot with a knob of butter for 5 minutes or until tender.

3. Salmon, peas, crème fraîche, and 50ml of water should be added. In the stock cube, crumble.
4. Stir in the chives and some black pepper after cooking for 3–4 minutes or until well heated through. To coat the spaghetti, continue stirring. Put food in bowls.

# Turkey Meatballs with Zoodles

Prep time: 10 minutes

Total time: 40 minutes

Serving: 2

## Ingredients

- 1 1/2 lb. zoodles
- Kosher salt
- 1/3 cup of plain breadcrumbs
- 1/4 cup of whole milk
- 8 oz. ground turkey
- 1/4 cup of ricotta
- 2 tablespoons of chopped fresh parsley
- 1 tablespoon of finely grated Parmesan
- 1/2 teaspoon of dried oregano
- Freshly ground black pepper
- Nonstick cooking spray
- 1 1/4 cups of jarred tomato sauce

## Instructions

1. In a large dish, toss the zoodles with plenty of salt. Let it settle for 10 minutes or until the zoodles start to soften and release some extra liquid. Dry them off and put them away.
2. In the meantime, mix the milk and breadcrumbs in a medium dish and set aside for approximately 5 minutes, or until the breadcrumbs soften and absorb most of the liquid. Using your hands, mix the breadcrumb mixture with the turkey, ricotta, parsley, Parmesan, oregano, 1/2 teaspoon of salt, and several grinds of black pepper. 12 meatballs should be formed.
3. 400°F should be the air fryer's temperature. Cooking sprays the inside of the basket, then add the meatballs, spacing them apart to allow for airflow. About

10 minutes into the air-frying process, flip the meatballs halfway through to ensure even browning on both sides.

4. Tomato sauce should be warmed up in a medium saucepan over medium heat in the meantime. Reduce the heat to low, stir in the meatballs, and keep warm.

5. Add several grinds of black pepper and 1/4 teaspoon of salt to the zoodles to season. Tossing halfway through, air fried for 5 to 6 minutes at 400 degrees F or until the food is soft and beginning to brown at the edges. Two dinner plates or shallow bowls should be divided between the zoodles, six meatballs, and warm tomato sauce. Serve with some Parmesan cheese on top.

# Smoky hake, beans & greens

Prep time: 15 minutes

Cook time: 10 minutes

Serving: 2

## Ingredients

- mild olive oil
- ½ x 200g pack of raw cooking chorizo
- 1 onion, finely chopped
- 260g bag spinach
- 2 x 140g skinless hake fillets
- ½ teaspoon of sweet smoked paprika
- 1 red chili, deseeded and shredded
- 400g can cannellini beans, drained
- juice ½ lemon
- 1 tablespoon of extra virgin olive oil

## Instructions

1. Heat the grill to high and bring a full kettle of water to a boil. In a large frying pan, heat 1 tablespoon of oil. Put the chorizo's flesh right in the pan after being squeezed out. After adding the onion, cook the beef for 5 minutes, breaking it up with a spatula until it is brown and covered with juices. Moreover, the onion will be tender and yellow.

2. Put the spinach in a colander and gradually pour the boiling water over it to wilt it before running it under the cold water faucet. Using your hands, squeeze out the extra water, then set it aside. Fish is placed on a baking sheet lined with foil,

which has been lightly greased. Add some seasoning, smoked paprika, and more oil before serving.

3.  Add the chili to the pan with the sausages and cook for an additional minute before adding the beans, spinach, lemon juice, and extra virgin olive oil. Gently reheat it before adding seasoning as needed.
4.  The fish doesn't need to be turned after grilling for 5 minutes or until flaky but not dry. Place a little amount of the bean mixture on each dish, then top it with the fish and any remaining liquids from the tray. If desired, top with a dollop of quick garlic mayo when serving.

# Sun-Dried Tomato & Arugula Lentil Salad

Prep time: 5 minutes

Cook time: 25 minutes

Serving: 2

## Ingredients

- 1/2 cup of dry lentils
- 2-3 cups of arugula
- 1/2 cup of sun-dried tomatoes
- 1 cup of grape tomatoes
- 2 Tablespoon of crushed walnuts
- 2 Tablespoon of goat cheese crumbles
- 2-4 Tablespoon of Vegan Turmeric Ginger Dressing

## Instructions

1.  As directed on the box, prepare the lentils.
2.  The arugula is topped with goat cheese, walnuts, halved grape tomatoes, sun-dried tomatoes, and dressing.
3.  Enjoy adding cooked lentils to your salads!

# Stir-Fried Chicken with Broccoli & Brown Rice

Prep time: 10 minutes

Cook time: 20 minutes

Serving: 2

## Ingredients

- 200g trimmed broccoli florets, halved
- 1 chicken breast, diced
- 15g ginger, cut into shreds
- 2 garlic cloves, cut into shreds
- 1 red onion, sliced
- 1 roasted red pepper from a jar, cut into cubes
- 2 teaspoons of olive oil
- 1 teaspoon of mild chili powder
- 1 tablespoon of reduced-salt soy sauce
- 1 tablespoon of honey
- 250g pack of cooked brown rice

## Instructions

1. Next, place the broccoli in a medium pan and bring it to a boil in the kettle. After covering the broccoli with water, boil it for 4 minutes.
2. In a nonstick pan that has been heated with olive oil, stir-fry the ginger, garlic, and onion for two minutes before adding the mild chili powder. Stir-fry the chicken for 2 more minutes after adding it. Save the water after draining the broccoli. Add the broccoli, soy sauce, honey, red pepper, and 4 tablespoons of broccoli water to a skillet and sauté until cooked through. Rice should be heated according to the directions on the package before serving with the stir-fry.

# Healthy Chicken Katsu Curry

Prep time: 20 minutes

Cook time: 35 minutes

Serving: 2

## Ingredients

- 25g flaked almonds
- 1 teaspoon of cold-pressed rapeseed oil
- 2 boneless, skinless chicken breasts
- lime wedges for squeezing over

*For the sauce*

- 2 teaspoons of cold-pressed rapeseed oil
- 1 medium onion, roughly chopped
- 2 garlic cloves, finely chopped
- a thumb-sized piece of ginger, peeled
- 2 teaspoons of medium curry powder
- 1-star anise
- ¼ teaspoon of ground turmeric
- 1 tablespoon of plain wholemeal flour
- For the rice
- 100g long-grain brown rice
- 2 spring onions, finely sliced

*For the salad*

- 1 medium carrot, peeled
- ⅓ cucumber, peeled
- 1 small red chili, finely chopped
- juice ½ lime
- a small handful of mint leaves
- a small handful of coriander leaves

## Instructions

1. Set the oven to 220C. For 35 minutes or until extremely soft, cook the brown rice in plenty of boiling water.

2. Sprinkle the almonds over a plate after crushing them in a mortar and pestle or until they are finely minced in a food processor. A little of the oil should be used to grease a small baking pan. The leftover oil should be used to season the chicken thoroughly on both sides. On the tray, cover the chicken with the nuts. Any leftover nuts from the platter should be pressed onto every breast. Bake for 20 minutes or until golden brown and well cooked. Slice thickly after resting for 4-5 minutes on the tray.

3. Make the sauce while you wait. The onion, garlic, and ginger are added to the hot oil in a medium nonstick saucepan. When gently cooking for 8 minutes or until softened and lightly browned, loosely cover the skillet and stir regularly. During the final two minutes, remove the cover, but watch out for burning the garlic.

4. Add the curry powder, star anise, turmeric, and plenty of freshly ground black pepper. Stirring occasionally, and continue cooking for a short while. Add the flour and whisk thoroughly. While continually stirring, gradually add 400ml of water to the pan.

5. The sauce should boil for 10 minutes while being stirred now and again. Cover loosely with a lid if it starts to sputter. After taking the pan from the heat, puree the sauce with a stick blender until extremely smooth. When needed, adjust the seasoning. Remain warm.

6. Add the spring onions and simmer for an additional minute once the rice is tender. Rinse well and let the pasta stand while you prepare the salad for a few minutes. Mix the cucumber and carrot with the herbs, lime juice, and chili.

7. Serve the rice, salad, and lime wedges for squeezing over, along with the sliced chicken between two dishes, followed by the sauce.

# Healthy roast dinner

Prep time: 15 minutes

Cook time: 50 minutes

Serving: 2

## Ingredients

- 285g medium potatoes, thickly sliced
- 4 small carrots halved lengthways
- 2 x 80g red onions, cut into quarters
- 170g large Brussels sprouts, trimmed
- 2½ teaspoons of rapeseed oil
- 2 teaspoons of thyme leaves
- 2 teaspoons of balsamic vinegar
- 1 large garlic clove, finely grated
- 2 pinches of English mustard powder
- 170g thick, lean fillet steak
- ½ teaspoon of vegetable bouillon powder

## Instructions

1. Oven temperature set at 180°C/160°F fan/gas 4. Cook the potatoes for 5 minutes in a big pan of boiling water. Save the water by draining.
2. Use 2 teaspoons of the oil to coat the potatoes, carrots, onions, and sprouts. A nonstick baking sheet should be used for the arrangement. 30 minutes of roasting after scattering with 1 teaspoon of thyme and some freshly ground black pepper.
3. Mix 1 teaspoon of the vinegar, the garlic, the remaining thyme and oil, the mustard, and a generous amount of black pepper as you wait. On a shallow plate, place the steak and rub this mixture over it. Mix the bouillon, 125 ml of the water you put aside in step 1, and the remaining vinegar, then set aside. After 30 minutes, flip the vegetables over and roast them for a further 15 minutes.
4. Over medium-high heat, preheat a small nonstick frying pan. Remove the steak from the marinade, brush out the extra, and fry for 2-3 minutes on each side or until done to your preference. Go to a board and relax there. The remaining marinade should be poured into the frying pan and cooked until it becomes somewhat thicker and gravy-like. Assemble the roast vegetables and gravy, slice the meat, and serve.

# Lemon Chicken

Prep time: 10 minutes

Cook time: 45 minutes

Serving: 6

## Ingredients

- 3 to 4 lb. chicken parts
- 4 teaspoons of lemon zest
- 1/3 cup of lemon juice
- 2 cloves garlic, crushed
- 2 tablespoons of fresh chopped thyme
- 2 teaspoons of fresh chopped rosemary
- 1 teaspoon of kosher salt
- 1 teaspoon of black pepper
- 2 tablespoons of butter, melted
- Lemon slices for garnish

## Instructions

### Marinate chicken:

1. In a large, non-reactive bowl, mix the lemon juice, lemon zest, garlic, thyme, rosemary, salt, and pepper.
2. Each chicken piece should have a thin 1/2-inch slice made into the underside using the point of a sharp knife.
3. Turn the bowl with the chicken pieces inside to evenly distribute the marinade. Put in the fridge and marinate for a couple of hours.
4. Lemon-Zest-Marined, Uncooked Chicken.

### Place chicken in the baking dish, and brush with butter:

1. Set the oven to 425 °F. Place the chicken, skin side up, in a single layer in a large baking dish after removing it from the marinade. Keep the marinade on hand. Melted butter should be applied with a pastry brush to each piece of chicken.
2. Lemon Chicken with Butter Brush in Baking Dish.

### Bake and baste with marinade:

1. After 20 minutes of baking, thoroughly basted the chicken pieces with the marinade that was saved. Bake the chicken for a further 15 to 25 minutes (a total of 35 to 45 minutes), or until the skin is crispy golden and the juices flow clear.
2. If you are cooking a variety of chicken parts, bear in mind that the breasts may be done before the thighs depending on their size, so you may need to remove them from the oven before the thighs.
3. After taking the chicken out of the oven, it should rest for 10 minutes in foil before being served.
4. Juices from the pan should be poured into a serving basin. To remove the fat off the surface, use a tablespoon of.
5. Serves the chicken with the liquids either on the side or drizzled over the top.

# Roast dinner for one

Prep time: 10 minutes

Cook time: 35 minutes

Serving: 1

## Ingredients

- 2 tablespoons of olive oil
- 1 large chicken breast, skin on
- 6 small new potatoes
- 2 carrots, cut into rounds
- 1 small onion, cut into wedges
- 3 broccoli spears or florets
- 3 thyme sprigs
- 1 bay leaf
- 150ml chicken stock, warmed
- ½ tablespoon of plain flour

## Instructions

1. Preheat to 200°C/180°F/gas 6 Season the skin of the chicken after applying 1 tablespoon of oil. Together with the thyme and bay leaf, place the potatoes, carrots, onion, and broccoli in a small roasting pan. Pour the remaining oil over everything, season it thoroughly, and toss to coat. Place the chicken breast on

top and roast for 25 to 30 minutes, or until the chicken is done and the vegetables are soft.

2. As you prepare the gravy, remove the chicken, potatoes, and broccoli from the roasting pan and set them aside. Add the stock to the tin and place it over high heat on the stove. Bring to a boil before simmering for a short while. To avoid any lumps, add the plain flour and whisk continuously. Turn off the heat after the sauce has thickened.

3. At an angle, cut the chicken breast into three to four pieces. Serve with gravy, potatoes, broccoli, and carrots.

# Chinese Chicken and Broccoli

Prep time: 15 minutes

Cook time: 10 minutes

Serving: 4

## Ingredients

### For marinating the chicken:

- 20 oz. skinless, boneless chicken breast
- 3 tablespoons of water
- 1 tablespoon of Shaoxing cooking wine
- ½ teaspoon of Kosher salt
- ¼ teaspoon of baking soda
- 2 tablespoons of cornstarch
- 1 tablespoon of oil any neutral oil is fine

### For the stir-fry sauce:

- ⅔ cup of soy sauce light sodium
- ⅔ cup of water
- 4 tablespoons of granulated sugar
- 2½ tablespoons of cornstarch
- 1½ teaspoon of toasted sesame oil

### For the rest of the dish:

- 1 lb. broccoli cut into florets
- 1½ tablespoons of garlic minced

- 1½ tablespoons of ginger minced

## Instructions

### *Marinate the chicken:*

1. The sliced chicken breast, water, Shaoxing rice wine, salt, and baking soda should first be mixed in a mixing dish. When the chicken has absorbed the majority of the liquids, mix thoroughly.
2. After that, stir in the cornstarch to thoroughly coat the chicken pieces. Add the oil to the marinade to complete it. Mix thoroughly and uniformly. As you prepare the remaining ingredients, set the chicken aside to marinate for 10 to 15 minutes or marinade it overnight.

### *Prepare the sauce:*

1. Mix all of the sauce's components in a dish or big measuring cup. Stir thoroughly until there are no more cornstarch clumps to be seen. Put aside till required.
2. Use an additional 1 to 2 tablespoons of cornstarch for a richer sauce if you want.

### *Make the chicken and broccoli:*

1. Broccoli florets are added to a kettle of boiling water. Depending on how tender you want your broccoli, cook it for anywhere from 30 seconds to 3 minutes. The size of the broccoli florets will also affect how long to boil them. Drain the cooked broccoli, then set it aside.
2. We often boil broccoli for one minute because we want it to be crisper.
3. Add enough oil to a wok or sauté pan over medium-high heat to cover the bottom thoroughly. When the oil is heated, add the marinated chicken and fry it until it is fully cooked on both sides. Take out of the wok or pan and place aside.
4. While it's not necessary, you may sear the chicken until it's golden brown if you'd like. Be careful to divide the chicken so that it cooks evenly, and if necessary, cook it in small batches.
5. Maintain medium heat and maintain 2 tablespoons of oil in the pan. If required, drain any extra oil. Add the minced garlic and ginger, and cook for 15 to 30 seconds or until fragrant.
6. Pour the stir-fry sauce into the pan with the garlic and ginger after giving it a thorough stir. Let the sauce heat up until it begins to simmer and the sauce becomes glossy and thickened. To keep the sauce from burning on the bottom, stir it regularly.

7. Reduce the heat to low, add the chicken, and stir in the broccoli florets after the sauce is uniformly thick and glossy. Stir until the sauce is well distributed throughout.
8. Enjoy when still hot and with rice!

# Mapo Tofu

Prep time: 10 minutes

Cook time: 10 minutes

Serving: 2

## INGREDIENTS

- 450 g soft tofu
- 100 g minced meat-beef or pork
- ½ tablespoon of sesame oil
- ½ teaspoon of salt
- 3 tablespoons of cooking oil, divided
- 1.5 tablespoons of Doubanjiang
- ½ tablespoon of fermented black beans
- 1 tablespoon of pepper flakes
- water or broth for braising
- 1 tablespoon of light soy sauce
- 1 teaspoon of sugar,optional for reducing the spiciness
- 2 finely chopped scallion whites
- 4 finely chopped garlic greens or scallion greens
- 2 finely chopped garlic cloves
- 5 finely chopped ginger slices
- ½ tablespoon of Sichuan pepper

### Water starch

- 2 and ½ tablespoons of water
- 1 tablespoon of cornstarch

## Instructions

1. Pork or beef mince should be lightly salted and peppered. Mix well and reserve.

2. Make cubes of square tofu (around 2cms). Add a pinch of salt after bringing a lot of water to a boil. Cook the tofu for one minute after sliding it in. Go away and drain. This aids in removing the taste of raw soy from tofu.

3. Get a wok, heat around 2 teaspoons of oil, and then fry the minced pork until it is crispy. Leave the oil in and remove it.

4. Then, add the fermented black beans, garlic, scallion white, and ginger and simmer for an additional 30 seconds to release their scent. Add another 1 tablespoon of vegetable cooking oil and fry the doubanjiang for 1 minute over low heat until it turns red (bringing us a gorgeous red color dish). Mix with some optional pepper flakes. As pepper flakes have little water and are quickly burned, they should be applied last.

5. Pour in some stock or water. Once the broth boils, add light soy sauce, sugar, and half of the cooked meat (to add extra flavor to the soup). Let it simmer for an additional 2-3 minutes. Add the tofu and cook for an additional 6 to 8 minutes. The tofu is better able to absorb the flavors due to the prolonged cooking period.

6. While the mixture is simmering, prepare water starch by combining 1 tablespoon of cornstarch with 2.5 tablespoons of water in a small bowl. Pour half of the mixture into the simmering saucepan after stirring the water starch. After about 30 seconds of back pushing and waiting, pour the remaining half. If the tofu isn't sufficiently salty, you can give it a faint taste and add a pinch. Add cooked beef to give the dish some crunch, and then pour sesame oil over it. Mix thoroughly.

7. When virtually all of the spices have adhered to the tofu cubes, remove them. Add chopped garlic greens and Sichuan peppercorn powder, if desired.

8. Steamed rice should be served right away.

# Hearty Asian Lettuce Salad

Prep time: 5 minutes

Total time: 20 minutes

Serving: 2

## Ingredients

- 1 cup of ready-to-serve brown rice
- 1 cup of frozen shelled edamame
- 3 cups of spring mix salad greens
- 1/4 cup of reduced-fat sesame ginger salad dressing

## Instructions

1. Follow the instructions on the package to prepare the rice and edamame.
2. Salad greens, rice, and edamame should all be mixed in a big dish. Add salad dressing and toss to mix. On two plates, divide the salad mixture and garnish it with the orange segments, radishes, and almonds.

# Prawn & Harissa Spaghetti

Prep time: 5 minutes

Cook time: 15 minutes

Serving: 2

## Ingredients

- 100g long-stem broccoli, cut into thirds
- 180g dried spaghetti, regular
- 2 tablespoons of olive oil
- 1 large garlic clove, lightly bashed
- 150g cherry tomatoes, halved
- 150g raw king prawns
- 1 heaped tablespoon of rose harissa paste
- 1 lemon, finely zested

## Instructions

1. Bring to a boil some water that has been mildly seasoned. Boil the broccoli for 1 minute 30 seconds, or until it is soft. Drain then set apart. Cook the pasta

according to the directions on the package, then drain, saving a ladle of the cooking water.

2. Add the garlic clove to a big frying pan with hot oil and cook for two minutes on low heat. Using a slotted spoon, remove and throw away, keeping the flavored oil.
3. The tomatoes should be added to the pan and fried for five minutes at medium heat or until they start to soften and become juicy. Add the prawns in with a stir, and cook for 2 minutes or until pink. While stirring, add the harissa and lemon zest.
4. Mix the prawns, harissa, and cooked spaghetti with the pasta water. Add the broccoli in with a stir, then season as needed and serve.

# Honey & Mustard Chicken Thighs with Spring Vegetable

Prep time: 10 minutes

Cook time: 40 minutes

Serving: 2

## Ingredients

- 1 tablespoon of honey
- 1 tablespoon of wholegrain mustard
- 2 garlic cloves, crushed
- zest and juice 1 lemon
- 4 chicken thighs, skin on
- 300g new potatoes, unpeeled
- 1 tablespoon of olive oil
- 100g spinach
- 100g frozen peas

## Instructions

1. Heat the oven to 200°C. Honey, mustard, garlic, lemon zest, and juice should all be mixed in a small bowl. Season the chicken thighs before adding the marinade.
2. Place the fresh potatoes in the spaces between the skin-side-up chicken on a large baking sheet. Sea salt should be added after the potatoes have been

covered with oil. 35 minutes of roasting in the oven should result in caramelized and occasionally burnt chicken skin.

3. To the roasting pan, add the spinach and peas. Once the spinach has started to wilt, and the peas are heated and coated in the mustardy sauce, return the dish to the oven for an additional two to three minutes.

# Cajun Cabbage Skillet

Prep time: 10 minutes

Total time: 35 minutes

Serving: 2

## Ingredients

- 2 tablespoons of canola oil
- 8 oz. chicken andouille sausages, sliced
- 1 small yellow onion, thinly sliced
- Kosher salt
- 1/2 small head of green cabbage, cored, halved crosswise
- 1/4 teaspoon of crushed red pepper
- 2 cloves garlic, minced
- 3 tablespoons of apple cider vinegar
- 1 tablespoon of unsalted butter
- 1/2 small sweet-tart apple such as Gala or McIntosh
- 1 large scallion, thinly sliced
- Hot sauce for serving

## Instructions

1. Over medium-high heat, preheat a large cast-iron skillet or high-sided saute pan. To uniformly coat the pan, add the oil and swirl the pan. Sausage slices should be added in a single layer and cooked for 2 minutes or until browned on the first side. About 2 minutes after flipping, grill the other side until it is browned. Slices of sausage should be transferred to a bowl with a slotted spoon and left aside.
2. Over medium-high heat, add the onion, a splash of water, and a generous amount of salt. While cooking, use a wooden spoon or heatproof rubber spatula to scrape up any browned pieces from the pan's bottom. For 5 to 7 minutes, or until the onion is beginning to get soft and lightly browned in areas, cook,

stirring periodically. Cook the cabbage for 6 to 8 minutes, turning periodically until it is crisp-tender. Add the crushed red pepper and another sprinkle of salt. Add another splash of water if the pan ever feels dry.

3. Cook the garlic and cider vinegar together for approximately a minute, stirring often, until the vinegar has largely evaporated. Returning the sausage to the pan when the butter has melted and adding the apple, stir periodically for 3 to 4 minutes or until the apple slices are just starting to get soft.

4. Add the scallion and serve right now with spicy sauce on the side.

# Spiced chicken with rice & crisp red onions

Prep time: 10 minutes

Cook time: 20 minutes

Serving: 2

## Ingredients

- 2 boneless skinless chicken breasts
- 1 tablespoon of sunflower oil
- 2 teaspoons of curry powder
- 1 large red onion, thinly sliced
- 100g basmati rice
- 1 cinnamon stick
- pinch saffron
- 1 tablespoon of raisins
- 85g frozen pea
- 1 tablespoon of chopped mint and coriander
- 4 rounded tablespoons of low-fat natural yogurt

## Instructions

1. Heat the oven to 190 C. Add curry powder after brushing the chicken with 1 teaspoon of oil. Pour the remaining oil over the onion. In a roasting pan, arrange the chicken and onions in a single layer. When the meat is done, and the onions are crisp, bake for 25 minutes, tossing the onions halfway through.

2. Rinse the rice and then add it to a pan with saffron, cinnamon, salt, and 300 ml of water. Bring to a boil, give it a quick stir, add the raisins, and then cover. Add the peas halfway through and gently simmer the rice for 10 to 12 minutes or until it is cooked. Divide the rice between the two dishes, then add the chicken

and onions on top. Before putting the yogurt on the side, mix the herbs into it and season as needed.

# Vegan jambalaya

Prep time: 10 minutes

Cook time: 35 minutes

Serving: 2

## Ingredients

- 2 tablespoons of olive oil
- 1 large onion, finely chopped
- 4 celery sticks, finely chopped
- 1 yellow pepper, chopped
- 2 teaspoons of smoked paprika
- ½ teaspoon of chili flakes
- ½ teaspoon of dried oregano
- 115g brown basmati rice
- 400g can of chopped tomatoes
- 2 garlic cloves, finely grated
- 400g butter beans, drained and rinsed
- 2 teaspoons of vegetable bouillon powder
- large handful of parsley, chopped

## Instructions

1. In a large skillet over high heat, heat the oil. Fry the onion, celery, and pepper for 5 minutes, tossing periodically until they begin to soften and turn color.
2. Rice and spices are mixed, followed by tomatoes, water, and a can of tomatoes. Add the beans, bouillon, and garlic and stir. Once the rice has reached a simmer and absorbed the majority of the liquid, cook it covered for 25 minutes. When the cooking time nears a finish, watch the pan to make sure it doesn't boil dry; if it starts to catch, add a little more water. Serve hot after adding the parsley.

# Cajun spiced salmon

Prep time: 20 minutes

Cook time: 5 minutes

Serving: 2

## Ingredients

- 2 salmon fillets
- juice 1 lime
- pinch chili powder
- ½ teaspoon of ground cumin
- ½ teaspoon of smoked paprika
- ½ teaspoon of ground coriander
- pinch of soft brown sugar
- drizzle of sunflower oil
- steamed rice to serve

### *For the salsa*

- 1 ripe avocado, peeled and diced
- a handful of cherry tomatoes, quartered
- 2 spring onions, sliced
- juice 1 lime
- splash of olive oil
- bunch of coriander, half roughly chopped

## Instructions

1. Salmon should be placed in a bowl, covered with lime juice, and allowed to "cure" for five minutes. Mix the sugar and all the spices in the meantime. Take the salmon out of the lime juice and cover it fully with the spices.
2. High grill heat. Place the salmon on a greased baking sheet with the flesh side up. Grill the salmon for 5 minutes or until it is well cooked, and the edges are turning dark. Gently mix the ingredients for the salsa with the coarsely chopped coriander while the salmon is cooking. After the fish is finished cooking, serve it with some rice, salsa, and some coriander sprigs.

# Thai prawn & ginger noodles

Prep time: 15 minutes

Cook time: 15 minutes

Serving: 2

## Ingredients

- 100g folded rice noodles
- zest and juice 1 small orange
- 1½-2 tablespoons of red curry paste
- 1-2 teaspoons of fish sauce
- 2 teaspoons of light brown soft sugar
- 1 tablespoon of sunflower oil
- 25g ginger, scraped and shredded
- 2 large garlic cloves, sliced
- 1 red pepper, deseeded and sliced
- 85g sugar snap peas, halved lengthways
- 140g beansprouts
- 175g pack of raw king prawns
- handful chopped basil
- handful chopped coriander

## Instructions

1. Place the noodles in a bowl and cover them with boiling water. Put aside for 10 minutes of soaking. To prepare a sauce, mix the orange juice and zest with the curry paste, fish sauce, sugar, and 3 tablespoons of water.
2. Half of the ginger and half of the garlic is added to the hot oil in a big wok. Cook for one minute while stirring. Stir-fry for three more minutes after adding the pepper. Add the sugar snap peas, toss, and heat for a moment before adding the curry sauce. Add the prawns and beansprouts, and simmer until the prawns just turn pink. After draining, add the noodles, remaining ginger, and herbs to the pan. Serve the noodles after thoroughly mixing them with the sauce.

# Veggie Okonomiyaki

Prep time: 15 minutes

Cook time: 10 minutes

Serving: 2

## Ingredients

- 3 large eggs
- 50g plain flour
- 50ml milk
- 4 spring onions, trimmed and sliced
- 1 pak choi, sliced
- 200g Savoy cabbage, shredded
- 1 red chili, deseeded and finely chopped
- ½ tablespoon of low-salt soy sauce
- ½ tablespoon of rapeseed oil
- 1 heaped tablespoon of low-fat mayonnaise
- ½ lime, juiced
- sushi ginger to serve
- wasabi, to serve

## Instructions

1. The eggs, flour, and milk should be thoroughly mixed. Add the cabbage, pak choi, soy sauce, and half of the spring onions. Pour the batter into a small frying pan with hot oil. For 7-8 minutes, cook covered over medium heat. The okonomiyaki should cook for a further 7-8 minutes, or until a skewer put into it comes out clean, after being flipped onto a second frying pan.
2. In a small dish, mix the lime juice and mayonnaise. Place the okonomiyaki on a platter, top with the additional chili, spring onion, and, if using, sushi ginger, and sprinkle with the lime mayo. If desired, serve the wasabi separately.

# Mediterranean turkey-stuffed peppers

Prep time: 20 minutes

Cook time: 30 minutes

Serving: 2

## Ingredients

- 2 red peppers
- 1 ½ tablespoons of olive oil, plus an extra drizzle
- 240g lean turkey breast mince
- ½ small onion, chopped
- 1 garlic clove, grated
- 1 teaspoon of ground cumin
- 3-4 mushrooms, sliced
- 400g can of chopped tomatoes
- 1 tablespoon of tomato purée
- 1 chicken stock cube
- a handful of fresh oregano leaves
- 60g mozzarella, grated
- 150g green vegetables

## Instructions

1. Heat the oven to 190C. Remove the seeds, core, and stems from the peppers after cutting them in half lengthwise. Olive oil should be drizzled over the peppers after seasoning them properly. Roast for 15 minutes after placing on a baking sheet.
2. In the meantime, warm 1 tablespoon of olive oil in a large pan over medium heat. Stirring to break up the lumps as it cooks, pour the mince onto a platter.
3. After cleaning it, heat the remaining oil over medium-high heat. After cooking the onion, garlic, and mushrooms for a further 2-3 minutes, add the cumin.
4. Return the mince to the pan and stir in the tomato purée and chopped tomatoes. Add the stock cube crumbles and simmer for three to four minutes before seasoning with oregano. After removing the peppers from the oven, stuff them as full as you can with the mince. Add the cheese on top, and bake for a further 10-15 minutes or until the cheese begins to turn golden.
5. Serve the peppers beside a mound of your favorite blanched, boiled, or steamed greens after carefully sliding them onto a dish.

# Salmon Pesto Traybake With Baby Roast Potatoes

Prep time: 5 minutes

Cook time: 45 minutes

Serving: 2

## Ingredients

- 500g baby new potatoes, cut in half
- 1 teaspoon of olive oil
- 2 large courgettes
- 1 red pepper, cut into small chunks
- 1 spring onion, finely sliced
- 25g pine nuts
- 3-4 salmon fillets
- juice ½ lemon
- 1½ - 2 tablespoons of pesto

## Instructions

1. After 10 minutes of boiling, drain the potatoes. Oven: Preheat to 200°C/180°F/gas 6. Place the potatoes on a baking sheet after tossing them in the oil. For 20 minutes, roast. Place the courgette, pepper, spring onion, and pine nuts in the center of the tray, pushing the potatoes to one side. On the other side, place the fish. Lemon juice should be squeezed over the veggies and fish fillets. Put pepper on everything. After the salmon is fully cooked, spread pesto over each fillet and place the baking dish back in the oven for an additional 12 to 15 minutes.

# Mustardy salmon with beetroot & lentils

Prep time: 10 minutes

Cook time: 10 minutes

Serving: 2

## Ingredients

- 2 tablespoons of olive oil
- 1 tablespoon of wholegrain mustard
- ½ teaspoon of honey
- 2 salmon fillets
- 250g pouch of ready-cooked puy lentils
- 250g pack of ready-cooked beetroot
- 2 tablespoon of crème fraîche
- 1 small pack of dill, roughly chopped
- 1-2 tablespoons of capers
- ½ lemon, zested and cut
- 2 tablespoons of pumpkin seeds, toasted
- rocket to serve

## Instructions

1. Set the oven to 200C. Mix 1 tablespoon of oil, mustard, honey, and some spice. Spread the honey and mustard mixture all over the salmon fillets after placing them on a baking sheet. Put the lentils and beets in a casserole, add the remaining oil, and season as needed. Place both in the oven for 10 minutes to fully cook the salmon.
2. Mix the lentils with the crème fraîche, dill, capers, and lemon zest. Together with the salmon, serve the pumpkin seeds, lemon wedges for squeezing, and, if desired, a side salad of rocket.

# Gingery broccoli fry with cashews

Prep time: 15 minutes

Cook time: 10 minutes

Serving: 2

## Ingredients

- 320g head of broccoli, stalks and florets separated
- 40g cashews, roughly chopped
- 1 tablespoon of sesame oil
- 15g ginger, finely sliced
- 1 small red onion, finely chopped
- 1 red pepper, deseeded and cut into thin strips
- 1 large carrot, cut into thin strips
- 2 garlic cloves, thinly sliced
- 1 red chili, deseeded and finely chopped
- 1 tablespoon of tamari
- 1 lime, juiced and zested
- 7g chopped coriander, plus extra to serve
- 2 eggs, beaten

## Instructions

1. In a food processor, pulse the broccoli stems until they are finely chopped. To get a texture similar to rice, add the florets and pulse one more.
2. In a wok or frying pan, roast the cashews just until fragrant. Transfer to a platter and reserve. Ginger, onion, pepper, carrot, garlic, and chili are added to a skillet with hot oil. Stir-fry for 2-3 minutes or until beginning to brown; cover and simmer for an additional 2 minutes.
3. When all the vegetables are soft, add the broccoli and 3 tablespoons of water and stir-fry for 3 minutes. Tamari, lime juice and zest, coriander, and eggs should be added and stir-fried just long enough to set the eggs. If desired, garnish the dish with cashews, more coriander, and extra slices of chili.

# Chicken & New Potato Traybake

Prep time: 15 minutes

Cook time: 1 hour 15 minutes

Serving: 2-4

## Ingredients

- 3 tablespoons of olive oil
- 500g new potatoes
- 140g large pitted green olives
- 1 lemon, quartered
- 8 fresh bay leaves
- 6 garlic cloves, unpeeled
- 4 large chicken thighs
- bag watercress or salad leaves to serve

## Instructions

1. Heat the oven to 200°C, 180°F, or gas 6. Add the potatoes, olives, lemon juice, bay leaves, and garlic to a large roasting pan after pouring in the olive oil. Mix everything together to cover everything with oil and spread it evenly. Season and add the chicken thighs with the skin facing up.
2. After one hour of roasting, baste the meat with the pan juices. Place the roasting pan in the oven. Check the potatoes for doneness and the chicken to ensure it is cooked through after one hour. Return the dish to the oven for a further 15 minutes to crisp the skin.
3. Take the roasting pan out of the oven. Using the back of a spoon, crush the roasted garlic cloves, remove the skins, and mix the mashed garlic with the meat juices. Serve alongside watercress or your preferred salad greens.

# Steamed trout with mint & dill dressing

Prep time: 1 minute

Cook time: 25 minutes

Serving: 2

## Ingredients

- 120g new potatoes, halved
- 170g pack of asparagus spears
- 1 ½ teaspoons of vegetable bouillon powder
- 80g fine green beans, trimmed
- 80g frozen peas
- 2 skinless trout fillets
- 2 slices lemon
- For the dressing
- 4 tablespoons of bio yogurt
- 1 teaspoon of cider vinegar
- ¼ teaspoon of English mustard powder
- 1 teaspoon of finely chopped mint
- 2 teaspoons of chopped dill

## Instructions

1. Set the young potatoes in a pan of boiling water to simmer until they are ready. To make the spears of asparagus shorter, cut them in half, then chop off the tips from the ends. Pour the bouillon into a big nonstick skillet. Add the beans and asparagus, cover, and simmer for 5 minutes.
2. Place the fish and lemon slices on top of the peas in the pan. Recover the lid and cook the fish for a further 5 minutes, or until it flakes easily but is still moist.
3. In the meanwhile, mix the yogurt, vinegar, mustard powder, mint, and dill. Add a couple of tablespoons of the fish's cooking liquid. Serve the vegetables with any lingering pan juices and the fish and herb sauce on top, along with the potatoes.

# Vegetarian Stir-Fry with Broccoli & Brown Rice

Prep time: 10 minutes

Cook time: 20 minutes

Serving: 2

## Ingredients

- 200g trimmed broccoli florets
- 150g vegetarian chicken
- 15g ginger, peeled and shredded
- 2 garlic cloves, finely chopped
- 1 red onion, sliced
- 1 roasted red pepper, from a jar, cut into cubes
- 2 teaspoons of olive oil
- 1 teaspoon of mild chili powder
- 1 tablespoon of reduced-salt soy sauce
- 1 tablespoon of honey
- 250g pouch of microwaveable brown rice

## Instructions

1. Pour boiling water over the broccoli in a medium pan, then cook for 4 minutes.
2. In a nonstick pan that has been heated with olive oil, stir-fry the ginger, garlic, and onion for two minutes before adding the mild chili powder. Stir-fry the vegetarian chicken-style chunks for an additional two minutes. Save the water after draining the broccoli. Add the broccoli, soy sauce, honey, red pepper, and 4 tablespoons of broccoli water to a skillet and sauté until cooked through. Rice should be heated according to the directions on the package before serving with the stir-fry.

# Key West Chicken

Cook time: 1 hour 15 minutes

Serving: 4

## Ingredients

- ¼ cup of lower-sodium tamari
- 3 Tablespoon of honey
- 1 Tablespoon of grated orange zest plus 1/4 cup of fresh juice
- 1 Tablespoon of grated lime zest plus 2 Tablespoons of fresh juice
- 1 Tablespoon of canola oil
- ½ teaspoon of fine sea salt
- ½ teaspoon of black pepper
- 1 large shallot, finely chopped
- 2 medium garlic cloves, minced
- 4 boneless, skinless chicken breasts
- Chopped fresh flat-leaf parsley

## Instructions

1. In a big bowl, mix tamari, honey, orange juice, lime juice, lime juice zest, oil, salt, pepper, shallot, and garlic. Chicken should be added and coated. Cover and refrigerate for at least 30 minutes or up to an hour to allow flavors to mingle.
2. Grill should be heated to between 400°F and 450°F. Chicken should be taken out of the marinade and placed aside while the grill is heating up. In a small saucepan, add the marinade and heat to a simmer (approximately 3/4 cup). Stirring regularly, simmer for 3 to 4 minutes or until reduced to 1/2 cup. Get rid of the heat.
3. Put the chicken on greased grill grates and cook it, covered, for 12 to 15 minutes, or until a thermometer inserted into the thickest part of the chicken reads 165°F. Serve with orange and lime wedges after being transferred to a big platter. Garnish with parsley.

Printed in Great Britain
by Amazon